Dedicated

To You
The Menopausal Woman

As a thank you for buying this book we invite you to join our
Phytomones VIP online club. Receive free gifts, special offers
and useful tips and information. Share your experiences with
others online in our private members only group.
Simply scan the code above on your smartphone or visit
http://budurl.com/phytovip

Learn more about Phytomones.
Join our Facebook group
http://Facebook.com/Phytomone
Or visit our website at
www.phytomone.com

Copyright Information Page

A Phytomones Ltd Book

First published in USA by Phytomones Ltd
This edition published by Phytomones Ltd
Copyright © 2012 by Jane Atherton
All rights reserved worldwide.

ISBN 978-1477518724

Phytomones Ltd
Registered Office: 1st Floor, 2 Woodberry Grove
Finchley, London, N12 0DR

Menopause Secret Book Reviews

Nick Panay, (BSc, MRCOG, MFSRH) – Consultant Gynaecologist, Chairman of the BMS,
"I am delighted to endorse and recommend Jane's book. It is particularly pleasing when a member of the British Menopause Society puts her head over the parapet and addresses a sensitive subject with such passion and insight. The science is right. If you are serious at making the most of yourself, physically and emotionally, read it and act!"

Sara Moger, Chief Executive, British Menopause Society.
"Several million women are adversely affected by 'the change of life'. Post reproductive health is a key phase, both physically and emotionally, in a woman's life and one when she is particularly vulnerable to health, well-being and lifestyle concerns.
This pair of books would be a positive support for these several million women, and if only 1% get to read them they will definitely gain benefit. And so will many people in their lives – husbands, partners, family, friends and work colleagues. The many women who sail through menopause will also find much to interest them in these excellent books.
Highly recommended."

Menopause Secret

"At 51, I'm not quite menopausal but I can't be far away so "The Menopause Secret" made very interesting reading. I am determined to make things as easy as possible for myself when the time comes and I think forewarned is forearmed. I love the ideas this book has for getting through the menopause as naturally and easily as possible. Of course, I'm planning on not having any symptoms (LOL) but if they do occur I'll know what to do and this book will be my first port of call."
By J.Small

Menopause Secret

"Wanted to know what was happening to me & this book answered my queries. A friend has since told me to get myself down to the Doctors for some HRT, but this book has given me the courage to try to manage my symptoms through diet/lifestyle. Read it through, but will be dipping back in as & when I need reminders."
By Mrs Kay

THE MENOPAUSE
Secret

A Lady's handbook

CHAPTER FOUR

FORWARD

The Menopause Secret

Over the past 30 years or so you have gotten to know yourself quite well. You know how you react to certain situations, what makes you laugh, what makes you cry. You know which foods you like, what wine you enjoy, what little things irritate you and which you are prepared to overlook.

Well, all of this will probably change as you journey along the road toward menopause, and at times you will feel like some deranged woman has invaded your body and is making you do things you're not familiar with. She will make you angry or upset at the oddest things, her memory is awful, her mind wanders off and is reluctant to return, and she doesn't fit into any of your clothes!!

Has your 'inner goddess' turned into your 'inner demon?'

This ultimate lady's handbook is the perfect guide to help you find your 'lost goddess'. *The Menopause Secret* will answer many of your concerns and help resolve many of the symptoms you may be having, giving you the knowledge and understanding to make the most of yourself during the menopause.

This book will inform you, motivate you, organise you, inspire you and work its menopause magic on you, so you can live the rest of your life like it's the best of your life.

The information in this book is not intended as medical advice or to replace the care of your doctor. Our intent is to share our knowledge based on scientific research and experience. We encourage you to consult with your doctor on all matters relating to your health and to seek medical supervision before embarking on any dietary, drug, exercise or other lifestyle changes.

MEET THE AUTHOR

Jane Atherton

SAC Dip. Clinical nutritionist
I.T.E.C Aesthetician
Member of BMS Council

Hello!
I have worked in the health and beauty industry for some 30 years, gaining international qualifications in clinical nutrition, exercise, beauty therapy and cosmetic science.
After working for some of the top cosmetic houses in the UK, I moved to Asia, where in-between having my two wonderful daughters, Amber and Yasmin, I operated a nutritional clinic, as well as writing articles for various health and beauty journals for the expatriate community.
Around two years ago I started having various unfamiliar physical and emotional symptoms.
Hot flushes, sleepless nights and erratic periods were not things I was used to in my daily routine. At one stage it crossed my mind that I could be pregnant, and then my hypochondriac self, started to believe I might have some serious illness. So I went to see my doctor who very calmly informed me, that I was in fact going through the menopause. My first reaction was - *thank the lord I'm not pregnant,* my second was, *what! No, wait, surely this can't be happening yet. I'm too young to be that old!*

Once I had gotten over the relief of not being pregnant and the shock of now officially being of a 'certain age', a sense of renewed optimism crept in. It really felt like the beginning of a new chapter, a fresh start, a time to drop all the bad habits and take up new ones. This new phase was like a breath of fresh air and certainly not something to feel morose about.

Things were looking good again, and I needed to channel all of this new-found energy into something worthwhile. So I took the opportunity to adapt my many years of knowledge and expertise in diet, exercise and beauty, and adjust it all to meet the changing needs of our menopausal bodies. Now I will show you how you can apply it to your life to keep you fit and active for the years to come.

While researching this book I found that most of the information out there, was quite 'medically heavy' and far too in – depth. Of course, medical issues have to be covered and I have spoken to many doctors and consultants, who have very kindly shared their professional knowledge with me. But this is not a medical book – the focus is on total balance, not anatomy. Therefore, inside you will find information on how to understand the 'whole' you, and how you can accomplish a synergy of the mind, body and soul… This is
The Menopause Secret

Another issue that came to my attention during this time was the lack of specific skin care products to deal with my changing skin needs. We have a high concentration of oestrogen receptors in the face and this is where the symptoms of the menopause may be at their most visible. I was concerned the products out there were not addressing these needs.
With extensive research and my cosmetic background experience, I went on to develop the 'Phytomone ™' skin and spa therapy range, specifically designed for hormonally changing skin.
The advanced formulation resulted in a carefully selected blend of bio-active ingredients to feed and nourish the skin and address the deeper lines that were now starting to appear, without the need for surgery. A cocktail of vitamins, minerals and essential oils, all specifically required during this stage of life were also added. The result is an impressive, luxurious range of skin and body care products that will target the problems we are facing.
I hope you enjoy using them and I'm sure you will find them beneficial.

The Menopause Management System is home to our complete range of products that will help to enhance your life both during and after the menopause, including:

The Menopause Secret: A complete guide to managing the menopause based on my professional experience and knowledge.

Menopause 30 day Concierge Programme: Helps you to kick – start your new regime, is extremely motivational and includes a wealth of interesting tips and information that will last you a lifetime. Buy this book on amazon.

Phytomone™: Advanced Spa therapy range for hormonally changing skin.

Nutritional supplements: Specifically targeted for the menopause. Our nutraceuticals will ensure beauty on the inside as well as the outside.

Home enhancing accessories: Decorate your home with our ultimate range of accessories. Indulge your sense of smell with our exotic candles, incense, pomanders, room sprays and linen sprays.

Clothing line: Our luxury range of leisure clothes uses the finest bamboo fibres to help absorb excess moisture, and will keep you feeling fresh and comfortable all day.

We would appreciate your feedback at http://phytomone.com

INTRODUCTION

Welcome to 'Part Two' of your life, ladies, and the Menopause Experience.

Every woman is going to experience her transition through menopause differently. The lucky few may sail through it and not have any symptoms at all, but most of us, by the time we hit 45-50 will be experiencing all that menopause has to offer with varying degrees of intensity.
It wasn't so long ago that women didn't live much beyond the menopause years, but how things have changed since our great-grandmothers day. We now have a wealth of information available to us at our fingertips, which has brought with it a new era of drugs to help improve our health and the quality of our lives. Indeed, we can look forward to living for at least another 20 or 30 years beyond the menopause. Statistics tell us that on average a woman lives until she is 82 and she will probably have her last period around the age of 51. This equates to approximately 1/3rd of your life being post – menopausal. So, as you can see, you still have quite a lot of living left to do.
We hope to help you get through the menopause transition with the least possible disruption. By giving you the knowledge and information that you need to make the right choices, we will show you how to minimise many of the symptoms you may be suffering from. By doing so, you will also be helping to prepare your body for the post – menopausal years ahead, ensuring you are in the best possible health for the rest of your life.

However, there are still many unanswered questions about the menopause, and new research brings with it an array of conflicting evidence. Hormone replacement therapy, the possible dangers of oestrogen dominance, benefits of progesterone and even the good old hot flush are all topics that are still up for debate in the medical industry. Science still has a long way to go before we understand completely why menopause happens.
But one thing we do know for sure is, it's a female fact of life and we are all going to go through it…

You may be oblivious to your initial stages of menopause, putting the weight gain down to a few too many glasses of wine, or you may think the hot flushes are due to some tropical disease you picked up on holiday last year. But you will have your moment of clarity and you will probably go through a whole array of emotions, just like I did. You may even feel a little sad because your days of reproducing are coming to an end, not because you want any more children at this stage of your life, but having the choice taken away from you may leave you feeling angry and empty. After all we are designed to reproduce, and not being able to because we're too old, can compound the feeling that everything has turned upside down. We are not ready to join the "Menopause Club" just yet, we want to stay young and vibrant.

Well, hold onto your hats because you have joined the biggest hormonal roller coaster ride in the park and this book is your ticket to help you enjoy it along the way!

Before we begin, it might help to know that you're not alone. There are around10 million women in the UK right now and around 50 million in America who are in some stage of the menopause. Luckily for us, unlike previous generations, we now have the advantage of having more knowledge available to understand what is happening with our hormones and why we are getting upset over the slightest things that we used to be able to laugh off, or why we hate our husbands, hate sex and want to run away to Bali to find ourselves…..Sound familiar? Then read on.

As it turns out, picking up this book may have been the hardest obstacle to overcome, but you've done it and you are on your way to accepting the fact that ageing and the menopause doesn't have to mean feeling or acting old. This is a time to live your life to the fullest, this is your 'new beginning' and you are not going to let your hormones hold you to ransom.

If you have become complacent over the years, as most of us do and have not been exercising as much as you should, or not paying much attention to your diet and lifestyle, then this could be just the gentle nudge you need to get you going. After all there is not much point living to a grand old age if it's full of pain and ill health. It wouldn't be much fun living life on the side – lines either.

So don't get your slippers and knitting out just yet and put the cocoa back in the cupboard, there is still far too much living to be done. This is definitely not your time to check out of life.

The aim of this book is to guide you through the stages of menopause, help you choose the right foods your body needs during this time of your life, and advise you on the types of exercise that are going to be most beneficial. We will also introduce you to the Phytomone range of products that have been specifically designed for hormonally changing skin and we will give your mind body and soul a make-over. You will be reminded how valuable life is and how to truly appreciate all it has to offer. It's easy to take so much for granted, especially where our health is concerned, but by the time you have finished reading you will have all the tools you need to create the perfect balance in your life. Make the changes now before it's too late. You won't regret it and you can look forward to living the rest of your life like it's the best of your life.

Look out for:
Menopause 30 day Concierge Programme

To help you make these changes and to ease you into your new way of life, we have developed the 'Menopause 30 day Concierge Programme' which is available to complement this book.

Why 30 days? – We have chosen 30 days because apparently this is the amount of time it takes for something to become a habit.
You will have 30 days of menus, easy to follow recipes and all of the help you need to stay motivated.

Each day you are given:

Meal Plan – A carefully chosen meal plan where the recipes have been specifically chosen to meet your body's changing needs, including calcium to maintain bone strength, phyto-oestrogens to help balances your hormones and an array of vitamins and minerals to help keep menopausal symptoms to a minimum.
Exercise Plan – A daily exercise plan that concentrates on your

requirements to help build bones, strengthen muscles and improve flexibility.

Exercise Tips – Extra tips to help keep you motivated along the way, and a range of supplementary bone- strengthening exercises that you can do anytime, anywhere.

Nutritional Tips – Includes interesting thoughts and ideas to help you get the most out of your eating plan and to encourage you to keep going.

Beauty Tips – We all know that true beauty comes from within, but glowing on the outside too will always lift your spirits. Use our daily beauty tips and make the best of yourself every day.

Body and Soul Tips –30 motivational thoughts and ideas to feed your soul and re-energize yourself.

Style Tips – Many tips and ideas to give you that 'put together' look without it being too stressful or expensive and restore your belief that you can look magnificent during menopause.

Take advantage of all the valuable information in this programme to develop new habits and bring about positive changes during your menopause transition, changes that your body now needs.

See our website for more details: http://phytomone.com

Chapter One

THE MENOPAUSE FACTS AND INFORMATION

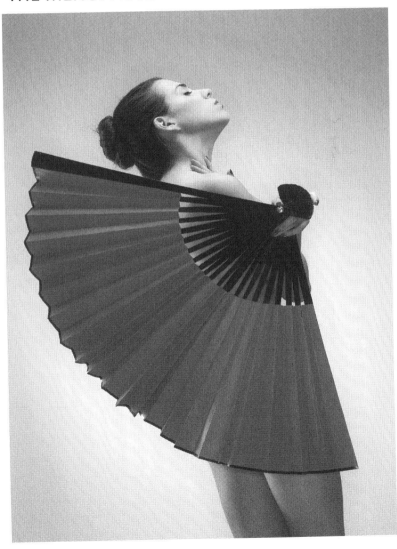

Not Sure If It's The Menopause?

Some women don't need any confirmation that they are going through the menopause and are quite happy to go with their instincts. However, if you are worried about anything or would simply feel more comfortable having your suspicions confirmed, then have a chat with your doctor who will be able to offer you a simple test to put your mind at rest. Alternatively you can purchase a home testing kit which is now widely available either in your local chemist or online. However, it is worth remembering that hormones do fluctuate throughout the month and although these tests can give you a good indication of what is happening they may not be 100 percent accurate.

Types of Hormone Tests

Some doctors may offer a blood test of your FSH levels to diagnose peri-menopause.. FSH stands for "Follicle Stimulating Hormone." During menopause high levels of this hormone are produced by the pituitary gland to try and stimulate the unresponsive ovaries, which decline over the years. High levels of FSH are a good indication that your ovaries aren't producing enough oestrogen, which is why your periods may have become irregular. The other hormone that can be measured is Luteinising Hormone (LH) also produced by the pituitary gland. It helps to increase the amount of oestrogen produced by follicle cells and stimulates ovulation. As your oestrogen levels drop, both of these hormones will be high, and this is a fairly good indication that you are in the early stages of menopause. But do bear in mind FSH levels can fluctuate throughout the month – so catch it at the wrong time of your cycle and you'll get a false reading.

Urine testing can be done either with your doctor or with home testing kits. Like blood tests they will measure your FSH levels, which, as mentioned before, can be highly variable throughout the month so may not give you an accurate reading.

Stages of Menopause

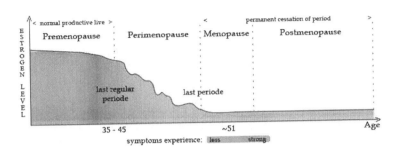

Peri-Menopause or Climacteric

This is where it all begins!

Peri-menopause literally means 'around menopause.' It is the transitional stage and refers to the time from which the hormone levels are changing up to when your periods stop. This phase can last anywhere between 2 to 10 years before complete cessation of the menstrual period, and usually begins between the ages of 35 and 50. During this phase symptoms may be non-existent, mild, moderate or severe and could last for months or years. It's difficult to give definitive information as every woman is unique and will experience peri-menopause differently.

Peri-menopause is most commonly characterised by irregular menstrual periods, hot flushes, night sweats, mood changes, depression, irritability, anxiety, nervousness and sleep disturbances including insomnia, loss of concentration, headache and fatigue.

Menopause

This stage represents the end of a woman's reproductive life. Oestrogen and progesterone production decrease permanently to very low levels, the ovaries stop producing eggs and a woman can no longer get pregnant naturally. Once you have gone 12 months without a period you are considered to be in menopause, and in fact, you will only be in the 'menopause stage' for a single day. Once the 12 months have gone by, you will then be 'post-menopausal'. It's worth noting that 90 percent of women who have not had a period for six months do not have another one.

Post Menopause

Refers to the stage of life after menopause has occurred. Once you have reached this stage you will be post-menopausal for the rest of your life. Many of the symptoms that occurred during peri-menopause will now become less frequent and intense and may stop altogether. However, the permanent decrease in oestrogen and progesterone levels can continue to affect your health, including a decrease in bone density, which can lead to osteoporosis. Bones may become weaker, making fractures more likely. During the first two years after menopause bone density decreases by about three to five percent each year, and after that by about one to two percent each year. You may also experience loss of muscle mass and strength and be subject to an increased risk of breast cancer. Other health problems due to low hormone levels include urinary tract infections, weak bladder, where small amounts of urine escape when laughing or coughing, decrease in the libido, and because the lining of the vagina becomes thinner and dryer, it may make sexual intercourse painful. Our skin also becomes thinner, dryer and less elastic due to the decrease in collagen, which is the protein that makes our skin young and supple. Fat levels increase and cholesterol levels rise, which may explain why atherosclerosis (blocked arteries) becomes more common among women after menopause. However, it is still unclear whether these changes are a result of ageing or a decrease in hormone levels. To help combat these problems, it is important to ensure you are in the best possible health by eating a healthy diet and following a regular exercise plan, that has been adjusted to suit your menopausal needs.

Hormones – Where They Come From and What They Do

There are many hormones in the human body but the group we're interested in are the 'steroid hormones', which include the sex hormones.

The steroid hormones are made from cholesterol in the adrenal glands and ovaries. Without enough cholesterol we cannot make sufficient steroid hormones, which is why it is important not to go on a no-fat diet (cholesterol is a type of fat produced by the liver).

Although the body is capable of manufacturing sufficient amounts of cholesterol, it is important not to cut it out of our diet completely. It can be found in foods such as poultry, fish, milk products, and egg yolks. Cholesterol is not found in foods of plant origin such as fruits, vegetables, grains, nuts, seeds, and dry beans and peas.

The steroid hormones affect all parts of the body including the brain, bones, circulation, digestion, liver, kidneys, nerves, muscles, reproductive organs and the immune system.
They are all intimately related to each other, each one being made from another, or turned back into another. From cholesterol, mitochondria, which are the cells power producers, make a hormone called Pregnenolone, which can then be transformed into progesterone or 17-OH-pregnenolone. All the other steroid hormones can then be made, depending on the body's needs including:

Testosterone
Predominantly a male sex hormone but also found in smaller amounts in the ovaries. Precursor to oestrogen and is also converted into oestrogen in your brain and around your heart. So you still have some naturally produced oestrogen in your body after the menopause.

Oestrogen
Female sex hormones that include estradiol, estriol and estrone. Collectively they are responsible for growth of female characteristics and regulating the menstrual cycle. Made primarily in the ovaries but also found in fat cells, muscle cells, and skin even after menopause.

DHEA (Dehydroepiandrosterone)
Precursor to the androgens, testosterone and oestrogen. Made in adrenal glands and declines dramatically as we age. Beneficial for immune system, memory and moods.

Corticosterone, Cortisol
Made in adrenal glands, helps to regulate numerous bodily functions including glucose and energy balance, moderate inflammation and immune responses.

The brain is the master switch that regulates hormone levels. The specific areas of the brain that control hormone levels are the hypothalamus and the pituitary glands.

Hormone imbalance disrupts signals to the brain and the hormone producing glands, which cause many menopausal symptoms and imbalances in our emotional state.

For example, testosterone, in excess, stimulates anger and aggression; whereas oestrogen in excess can stimulate over-sensitivity and a deficiency may cause depression. DHEA can stimulate a feeling of well-being and progesterone promotes feelings of calm.

Merry Little Dance of The Hormones

If you cast your mind back I am sure you will remember the emotions you experienced when you were going through puberty; you must recall the mood swings, tender breasts, blemishes and emotional outbursts just before your period started. This was your body preparing for your reproductive years by turning on your hormones. Well, going through the menopause is sort of like going through puberty, only in reverse. You are now coming toward the end of your reproductive years and your body is preparing to switch your hormones off by slowly producing less oestrogen and progesterone.

Unfortunately, when our hormones perform this merry little dance, they do so in quite an erratic fashion, with spikes and falls throughout the month, resulting in many of the menopausal symptoms.

There is no doubt that peri-menopause can be stressful at times, but there is light at the end of the tunnel, you just need to hang on in there while it's happening. Once you finally make it to the menopause stage, your hormones will start to settle down and your symptoms will be less severe. Your hot flushes will decrease, and your sleeping patterns should return to some form of normality, bringing higher energy levels and a clearer mind, which hopefully will put some 'zest' back into your life. Aching muscles should ease and mood swings become less severe.

The post menopause feeling will give you a new sense of freedom.

You no longer have to worry about birth control, and finally, after 30 years or so, you can now look forward to a life without having a monthly period. At long last you have your body back; it is no longer available for puberty, periods, pregnancy or peri-menopause.

The sense of stability, both mentally and physically, that comes about after menopause is powerful and will give you a renewed sense of optimism, confidence and self-awareness This is your time, and it is up to you to make sure you take advantage of it all and enjoy your life to the fullest. Don't let it pass you by!

FSH – Follicle Stimulating Hormone

As mentioned earlier, this hormone is produced in the pituitary gland at the base of the brain and it is the main hormone involved in producing mature eggs. But the eggs that now remain don't respond as well to FSH as they did when they were younger. As a result the ovaries will start failing to release eggs, which in turn reduces the production of oestrogen and progesterone. In an attempt to encourage the ovaries to respond, the pituitary gland releases more FSH into your bloodstream to try and stimulate the unresponsive ovaries. These high levels of FSH indicate that your ovaries are starting to fail. Your periods will probably become irregular and unpredictable as your hormone levels fluctuate, until they stop altogether.

You are born with all the eggs already in your ovaries; on average you will have between one to two million immature eggs or follicles, and will never produce anymore in your lifetime. Throughout your life, the vast majority of follicles will die through a process known as atresia. Atresia begins at birth and continues throughout the course of your reproductive life. When you reach puberty and start to menstruate, only about 400,000 follicles remain. With each menstrual cycle, a thousand follicles are lost and only one lucky little follicle will actually mature into an ovum (egg), which is released into the fallopian tube. If it is not fertilised it will be shed during your period. You will ovulate approximately 450 eggs in your reproductive lifetime. Even when pregnant you are still losing eggs. When you are about twenty-eight to twenty-nine years old, you will start to lose eggs a little faster. By the time you are thirty-five the rate of egg loss is much increased, and at forty, the rate of dying eggs is extremely rapid and falls to low numbers. At menopause relatively few or no eggs remain.

Oestrogen

This is not just one hormone as many people think, it's a group of female hormones produced in the ovaries, adrenal glands and fat cells. In an adult woman the three different oestrogens are:

Estradiol: Produced by the ovaries; it is the most dominant oestrogen before menopause and is necessary for almost every function in the body and brain. Estradiol is responsible for good memory, high energy levels, good sex drive, smooth skin and cheerful outlook on life.

Estrone: Produced by the fatty tissues; it is less potent than estradiol but becomes more abundant after menopause when estradiol is reduced.

The more fat you have, the more estrone you make. It has been proven to increase risks of early heart attacks, reproductive cancers and diabetes.

Estriol: Prominent during pregnancy and made from a combination of components from the placenta, foetus and mother.

Oestrogen is responsible for regulating the function of reproduction in the female body; it regulates menstrual cycles and prepares the uterus for pregnancy. This hormone plays a key role in shaping the female body, particularly the breasts and hips, and is responsible for maintaining the health of the skin.

During the peri-menopause transition the ovaries gradually stop making oestrogen; this is a natural process and not a sign of illness. Levels can go up and down in quite an erratic fashion for years before the final cut off. These fluctuating hormone levels are thought to be behind many menopausal symptoms, such as hot flushes, fatigue and vaginal dryness, and could be a result of either the high or low levels of oestrogen in the body.

Although the production of oestrogen winds down at menopause, the ovaries continue to produce testosterone, which is converted into oestrogen in the liver and fat tissue – Women with a lot of fatty tissue, especially in their buttocks, abdomen and thighs, produce more of this hormone and thus have more oestrogen than thinner women do. This may be one reason why heavier women are at higher risk of breast cancer and other oestrogen-sensitive cancers.

There is no doubt that oestrogen is extremely beneficial. The key is to know when it becomes the dominant hormone because this is when it becomes toxic to the body.

Symptoms of Oestrogen Dominance

- Autoimmune disorders
- Allergies
- Bloating
- Breast cancer
- Cervical dysplasia
- Depression
- Fatigue
- Hair Loss
- Headaches
- Increased blood clotting
- Irregular menstruation
- Irritability
- Insomnia
- Loss of libido
- Memory loss
- Mood swings
- Osteoporosis
- Polycystic ovaries
- Premenopausal bone loss
- PMS
- Thyroid dysfunction
- Uterine cancer
- Uterine fibroids
- Weight gain

Symptoms of Oestrogen Deficiency

- Hot flushes
- Rapid pulse rate
- Bloating
- Dry skin
- Vaginal dryness
- Fatigue
- Poor memory
- Joint pain, swelling and stiffness
- Osteoarthritis
- Loss of libido
- Depression
- Headaches
- Unexplained weight gain
- Low back pain

Oestrogen and Cancer

Although oestrogen does not appear to directly cause cancer. It is caused by DNA damage, or mutations, which could have been either inherited or caused by chemicals such as those found in cigarette smoke. The mutations can occur spontaneously, as a result of mistakes that were made when a cell duplicates its DNA molecules prior to cell division.

If the cells are damaged they are at more risk of becoming cancerous and it is oestrogen's ability to stimulate cell growth, particularly in hormone-sensitive tissue such as the breast and uterine lining, that makes excess oestrogen in the body such a dangerous promoter of cancer.

Out of the three oestrogens, estradiol is the most stimulating to the breasts and estriol the least. Synthetic ethinyl estradiol, which is commonly used in oestrogen supplements and contraceptives, is even more of a risk for breast cancer because it is absorbed by the mouth and slow to be metabolised and excreted. The longer a synthetic oestrogen stays in the body, the more opportunity it has to do harm.

Xeno-oestrogens
Environmental Oestrogens

Not heard of them before? Don't worry most people haven't, but it's important for all of us to be aware of the effects of oestrogens in our environment. Environmental hormones can cause an imbalance of female hormones, creating a host of oestrogen dominance symptoms. Xeno-oestrogens, which literally means "foreign oestrogen," are man-made compounds mainly derived from petroleum oil and have the ability to mimic the effects of natural oestrogens in the body, which can increase our natural oestrogen levels over time. Petro-chemically based xeno-oestrogens are difficult to detoxify through the liver, so they stay in the body a lot longer.

Much of our world now revolves around the use of petroleum oil, including fuel for our machines and the manufacture of millions of products, such as clothing, foods, medicines, cosmetics, solvents and packaging. Synthetic oestrogens and progestins are also found in the urine of millions of women who take birth control pills and hormone replacement therapy, it is flushed away down the toilet and eventually works its way into the food chain. Oestrogenic drugs are also fed to the animals we eat to fatten them up. They in turn are passed onto us through our diet. The price we pay for having many of these conveniences in our lives today is pollution in our water, our soil, the very air we breathe, as well as in our bodies.

The effects of xeno-oestrogens on the environment and the detrimental effects they are having on the human body are still being studied, and the results may not show up until the next generation. What we do know for now, is that the on-going tests being done by scientists show, beyond doubt, that xeno-oestrogens are threatening the survival of many birds, reptiles and mammals. It is just a matter of time before we have proof of the danger they cause to humans. Although the amount of xeno-oestrogens we are exposed to is relatively small, and you may feel they are so diluted that there is little cause for concern, remember to take into account the multitude of ways in which we are exposed to these substances every day!

A Few Suggestions to Avoid Xeno-oestrogens

• Have a good water filter for your source of water.
• The growth hormones fed to cattle, pigs, poultry, and other livestock are another major source of xeno-oestrogens. Buy hormone free meats and dairy products where possible.
• Avoid plastic goods - they leach into the environment.
• Do not microwave food in plastic containers, and especially avoid the use of plastic wrap to cover food for microwaving.
• Use glass or ceramics whenever possible to store food.
• Avoid Teflon and other non-stick cookware. Cast iron is an inexpensive, durable, and healthful alternative.
• Do not leave plastic containers, especially your drinking water, in the sun.
• If a plastic water container has heated up significantly, throw it away - do not drink the water either. Try and use glass bottles where possible.
• Don't use fabric softeners as they put petrochemicals directly onto your skin where they can be readily absorbed.
• Use a simple laundry and dish detergent with less chemicals.
• Use organic soaps and toothpastes. Avoid fluoride.
• Xeno-oestrogens absorbed by the skin are ten times more potent than those taken orally, because they have the ability to travel directly to the tissues instead of passing through the liver. Avoid creams and cosmetics that have toxic chemicals and oestrogenic ingredients such as parabens, phenoxyethanol, and other compounds. Look out for them in body lotions, toothpastes, soaps, gels, hairsprays and shampoos. Switch to more natural products. Cheap brands usually have more toxic ingredients.
• Avoid nail polish and nail polish removers.
• Use only naturally- based perfumes. Most perfumes are petro-chemically based.
• Avoid surfactants found in many condoms and diaphragm gels.

Plastics, especially soft plastics, contain many compounds that are considered to be xeno-oestrogens. Phthalates, a type of plasticiser used to make plastics soft and flexible, are a common offender. These compounds can leach out over time in response to heat or other stimuli. Phthalates are used in many products including food storage containers, packaging, children's toys, certain clothing and footwear items, toiletries, pesticides, baby bottles... the list goes on and on.

Avoid all pesticides, herbicides, and fungicides. Wash your food well to get rid of the pesticides and buy organic wherever possible. The following crops have the highest residues of xeno-oestrogens:

- Strawberries
- Spinach
- Cabbage
- Pineapples
- Green Beans
- Asparagus
- Apricots
- Raspberries
- Cherries
- Apples
- Peaches
- Grapes
- Sweet Peppers

Phyto-oestrogens

Phyto-oestrogens (phyto meaning plant) are naturally occurring oestrogenic compounds that are found in a variety of plant foods such as beans, seeds, and grains. They have a similar structure to the hormone oestrogen and can bind to oestrogen receptors throughout the body mimicking the effects of oestrogen.
These compounds are generally weak oestrogens, in comparison to real oestrogen and can be beneficial to a woman if she is suffering from oestrogen deficiency. On the other hand anyone who is experiencing oestrogen dominance will likely want to avoid too many phyto-oestrogens where possible as they may contribute to the problem.

More about this can be found in the chapter on nutrition.

Progesterone

Progesterone is a master hormone; it is used as a precursor for the production of other important hormones, such as oestrogen, testosterone and cortisone. Progesterone affects every tissue in your body including the uterus, cervix and vagina, the immune system, water balance and bone cells, to name a few. This hormone is produced by the ovaries and helps to prepare the uterus for pregnancy. Levels of progesterone rise dramatically at ovulation and then fall significantly if fertilisation doesn't occur.

The decrease of progesterone levels at menopause is proportionately much greater than the decrease of oestrogen. On average oestrogen declines by 40 to 60 percent whereas progesterone can decrease to nearly zero.
Allowing oestrogen to dominate the hormonal environment could cause serious medical issues. Progesterone's job is to balance oestrogen levels. Some research points toward a lack of progesterone giving rise to many menopausal symptoms - rather than a lack of

oestrogen. Increasing progesterone levels with natural bio-identical progesterone could relieve many symptoms.

Natural Progesterone:
Produced by the ovaries after ovulation and by the placenta during pregnancy. Progesterone prepares the uterus for implantation of a fertilised egg and helps maintain pregnancy.

Bio-identical Progesterone:
Progesterone was discovered and isolated in the early 1930's. Initially this hormone was obtained from the ovaries of pigs and later from human placentas. Both these methods were expensive and only yielded small quantities of progesterone.

In 1938 an American biochemist, Russell E Marker manufactured progesterone in a laboratory by converting another substance, diosgenin found in the Mexican Wild Yam, into progesterone through a series of chemical changes. In soy the steroid substrate stigmasterol is converted into progesterone.

Since the 1940's they have been using soybeans, wild yams and other plants from the tuber family to make progesterone. Today, progesterone is produced for pharmaceutical purposes in the laboratory with the aid of an enzyme. Progesterone cannot be converted from wild yams or soybeans by the body.

In the early 1990's U.S. medical practitioner, Dr. John Lee M.D. pioneered and published books on the benefits of natural progesterone to manage menopausal symptoms, premenstrual syndrome and breast cancer. He discovered natural progesterone has a significantly more important action on the body than progestins (synthetic progesterone), which have an extremely limited action. Some information suggests that there is still a lack of understanding by mainstream medicine on the important difference between natural progesterone and the synthetic progestins, with some believing they both produce the same effects and results. This lack of understanding or disagreement on the subject has been the source of great controversy for many years in medical circles.

Progestins: Synthetic forms of progesterone that mimic most or all activities of progesterone, but do not have the same chemical structure. They are widely used in HRT and birth control pills. Natural bio-identical progesterone, used in doses no greater than the body would normally make, has virtually no side effects, whereas the synthetic progestins have many. Progestins are commonly synthesised from progesterone or another synthetic hormone called nortestosterone. They have some progesterone-like effects but they are not natural, meaning neither of them is found in nature. Unlike natural progesterone, progestins can result in an array of potential side effects such as joint and muscle pain, painful breasts, mood swings and weight gain. Progestins are not natural and are foreign to the human body. In addition to their potential for undesirable side effects, they fail to provide the full benefits of natural progesterone and can inhibit normal progesterone production and compete for progesterone receptors, thus, effectively blocking your own natural progesterone.

Progestogens: The term is used to describe hormones that provide progesterone-like activity, and this includes both progesterone and progestins.

If you are deficient in progesterone, using a natural bio-identical progesterone supplement cream in correct amounts may have very positive results for you and your menopausal symptoms. Progesterone is a highly fat soluble compound that is absorbed exceedingly well when applied trans-dermally, where it passes through the skin into the layer of fat that lies beneath, known as subcutaneous fat. The more progesterone deficient you are, the more readily it is absorbed. However, be aware that the results may be different if you use too much, or you are not truly progesterone deficient, because the benefits may then be lost or reversed. More is not better in this case. You are aiming for the amount your body would make if it was balanced, otherwise known as a physiologic dose.

At the moment progesterone cream is only available in the UK by prescription. A deficiency can be confirmed by your doctor.

Symptoms of Progesterone Deficiency

- Absence of menstruation.
- Loss of libido
- Mood swings
- Osteoporosis
- Increased risk of endometrial cancer
- Night sweats and hot flashes
- Breast tenderness
- Carbohydrate cravings
- Irregular periods
- Ovarian cysts
- Menstrual cramps
- Puffiness/bloating
- Water retention
- Lower body temperature

Symptoms of Progesterone Dominance

- Drowsiness
- Acne
- Mood swings and depression
- Weight gain
- Lower libido
- Headaches

Testosterone

One of the main male hormones, it is also produced by women in smaller amounts. This is one of the androgen, or male hormones, and is secreted by the ovaries and adrenal glands. Testosterone influences your energy levels, your libido, and helps maintain muscle and bone strength. At menopause this hormone starts to slow down, and after menopause we produce about half the amount we used to. This drop in testosterone causes muscle mass to decrease, which in turn lowers the metabolism and increases fat cell production, and the re-distribution of fat from our thighs and buttocks to the abdomen, hence the thicker waist and weight gain during menopause. It may also cause thinning of the hair or hair loss, and at the same time, cause the odd hair to grow in places we don't really want, such as the face and chest.

Menopause Symptoms
The Cause and The Cure

It is important to remember that these signs and symptoms of the menopause are temporary. This is what your body is meant to do to prepare you for the new role and lifestyle that doesn't involve childbearing. Menopause shouldn't be viewed as an illness and many of the symptoms can be minimised by adjusting your lifestyle. Your body is changing and therefore so must you.

Irregular Periods
One of the earliest symptoms of peri-menopause and an indication that your hormone levels are beginning to fluctuate. Your periods may become longer and heavier or shorter and lighter.

Cause: When your ovaries start running out of eggs, your hormone secretion becomes erratic. Some months you may ovulate and some you may not. Oestrogen levels can rise sharply and then drop, which means you may miss periods, or even have them more frequently with a heavier flow than usual during some months. Your periods are likely to become increasingly irregular and unpredictable before eventually stopping altogether. It's worth remembering that you can still become pregnant during this stage.

Cure: There is not really a cure for this. You are on the menopause merry-go-round, so try to enjoy the ride as much as you can and be prepared for the unexpected. Make sure you always keep a tampon or a sanitary pad in your bag when going out and some reserve in the bathroom cabinet. Keep track on your calendar and remember that over 90 percent of women who have not had a period for six months do not ever have another one.

Hot Flushes

Hot flushes are the hallmark of the menopause and a common symptom, with up to 75 percent of women suffering with them. They generally continue for about two years, but can carry on for many more. A hot flush is a feeling of intense heat generally spreading from your face, neck and chest and can last for several minutes. Your hot flush may also cause visible signs of facial flushing as the blood flow is redirected to the skin, and it is common to begin sweating. Immediately following a hot flush there can be a significant drop in body temperature and you may experience a chill afterwards. You may also experience rapid or irregular heart beat and pulse, including heart palpitations.

Cause: The exact reason for hot flushes and night sweats is still not fully understood and research is on-going. One theory is thought to be associated with the fluctuation in oestrogen levels and a rise in the follicle stimulating hormone (FSH). This fluctuation confuses the hypothalamus, the body's thermostat, into thinking your body is too hot. The brain responds by sending out an alert that indicates a number of changes. Your heart pumps faster, the blood vessels in your skin dilate to circulate more blood to radiate off the heat, causing the 'flushed' effect, and your sweat glands release sweat to cool you off even more.
This in-built cooling mechanism is how our bodies stay cool in the summer, but during a hot flush it is mistakenly brought on by an imbalance of hormones. Low oestrogen levels are often blamed , but other studies have shown that women are oestrogen dominant 10 to 15 years prior to menopause, and instead of more oestrogen they need increased progesterone to rectify the problem. Studies carried

out by Helene Leonetti and published in the Obstetrics and Gynaecology Journal (1999) showed that not only hot flushes, but also many other menopausal symptoms, responded well to topically applied progesterone cream. So raising the levels of your progesterone could be all you need to control your hot flushes. Some women are more sensitive than others to this temperature change and may experience intense hot flushes throughout the day and night.

Cure: Start by recording your hot flushes on the calendar – As well as hormone imbalance, hot flushes may be compounded by things such as spicy foods, alcohol, caffeine, stress, smoking or something in particular you were doing at the time; if you can identify the specific trigger, you will have the opportunity to change your diet and lifestyle to try and manage your hot flushes, before you start to think about hormone replacement therapy, or any other medication such as anti-depressants.

Try wearing layers that can be easily removed and then replaced and have a small fan handy. Exercise is important; it vastly improves circulation and can make the body more tolerant of temperature extremes, and breathing exercises may also help combat the symptoms. If you find that lifestyle changes and the natural approach don't help and your hot flushes are impacting too much on your sleep or daily life, then you might want to talk to your doctor and consider alternative options such as a natural bio-identical progesterone cream or hormone replacement therapy.

Hot flushes usually start to decline about two years after menopause, but once again there is no guarantee of this.

Night Sweats

Are no fun at all and if they disturb sleep on a continual basis you can feel worn out and exhausted the next day.

Cause: The same as for hot flushes.

Cure: Sleep in cotton pyjamas or nightgown on cotton sheets, and keep an electric fan by your side of the bed, along with a damp face cloth. Avoid caffeine and alcohol and make sure your bedroom isn't too hot.
If you are oestrogen dominant then you may benefit from applying natural bio-identical progesterone cream before you go to sleep, to help raise your progesterone levels and bring about a balance of oestrogen and progesterone.

Natural Remedies

Regular exercise.
Deep Breathing exercises.
Sage – Make as a cup of tea, one tablespoon per cup and infuse for ten minutes. Sage is effective in cooling the blood.
Dong Quai – May help balance the pituitary gland. However, it can thin the blood and make skin more sensitive to the sun, so take precautions. Women should not take this if suffering from fibroids, haemophilia or other blood clotting problems.
Black Cohosh – A popular remedy, which contains plant hormones that can act as herbal hormone therapy, though its effectiveness remains unclear and there are some concerns with liver toxicity if used excessively. Avoid if you are oestrogen dominant.
Natural Bio-identical Progesterone Cream
In the UK you cannot buy natural progesterone cream over-the-counter like you can in many other countries, though it is available online or by prescription from your doctor. If using progesterone cream read the label very carefully and make sure it contains only natural bio-identical progesterone. Wild yam or soy will have no benefit at all on progesterone levels.

Some herbalists believe that the liver may contribute towards menopausal symptoms including hot flushes. Dandelion and milk thistle are particularly good for cleansing the liver; try drinking dandelion tea or adding a few drops of milk thistle tincture (5ml) to a glass of water.

Phytomone Spa Therapy Treatments
Designed with the menopausal woman in mind. These hormone balancing products may help alleviate your symptoms.
For hot flushes and night sweats we recommend the Cooling Body Powder or the Cooling Spray Gel to help absorb excess moisture and cool you down.

Weight Gain

Menopause can be responsible for about a 10 to 15 pound weight gain in most women, with up to 90 percent of menopausal women gaining some weight.
Much of this weight, approximately one pound per year, is gained during peri-menopause. As our oestrogen, progesterone and testosterone levels drop, it brings about a change in body shape, and fat starts to accumulate around your middle section rather than your hips and buttocks, making it feel like you have gained more weight as your waist bands start to feel tighter.

Cause: While it is true that diminished hormones cause us to gain weight and make it harder for us to lose, there are other factors that contribute. In reality, you have probably gained some weight in the years building up to menopause, and studies show that menopausal women are less inclined to exercise. As we age our metabolism slows down and our muscle mass diminishes, causing the composition of the body to shift to more fat and less muscle. Having more fat than muscle means your metabolic system burns fewer calories. So, if you continue to eat the way you have been doing you are likely to gain weight.
Testosterone, one of the androgen hormones, is the one that helps your body create lean muscle, and at menopause levels drop, causing a loss of muscle mass.
Fat cells also contain oestrogen and as our oestrogen levels drop our body is keen to hold on to as much oestrogen as it can, making it difficult for us to lose the weight.

Cure: You need to make changes in your lifestyle and commit to an exercise program. Take a look at your diet. You may think it is healthy and well balanced but is it really? Are you getting balanced portions of proteins, fats and carbohydrates? Read the chapter on nutrition to help you adjust your diet if necessary, or kick- start your regime with the 30-day concierge programme.

Mood Swings

During menopause women often experience mood swings because of their unbalanced hormones. These moods can be compounded by other menopausal symptoms such as disturbed sleep due to night sweats or insomnia, a dry vagina and weight gain.

Midlife is also a time when there can be other stressful life events going on such as problems with relationships or work pressure, issues with children, especially if they have reached puberty and have their own hormonal issues. This is also quite a common time for children to be leaving home and going to university, which in itself is worrying and can also leave you with that 'empty nest' feeling. There may be concerns about elderly relatives and how to take care of their health problems. So women in their forties and fifties can already have life changing issues going on, and all this comes at a time when your self-esteem and your perception of your body image is probably quite low.

Cause: Medical researchers have found that oestrogen seems to play a large role in the brain's production of serotonin, also known as the mood-regulating neurotransmitter. Because peri-menopausal hormone imbalances temporarily disturb serotonin production in the brain, there is an increased chance of mood swings, depression and other psychological disturbances during menopause.

Excess oestrogen can also have a negative effect on your mood as it can alter the copper and zinc ratios, causing the body to retain copper and lose zinc. Symptoms of excess copper include anxiety, depression, mood swings as well as achy joints, muscle pain and insomnia. A deficiency in zinc can cause fatigue, poor memory and blood sugar imbalance to name a few.

Cure: Sometimes just knowing why you are feeling like you do can be a relief. Try and keep things in perspective and tell yourself it is just a temporary feeling. Make a note on the calendar and see if there is anything specific that triggers your mood swings or if they come at certain times of the month, similar to PMS. In fact, women who experienced PMS are more likely to experience mood swings during menopause.

Your diet may be contributing to your mood swings. Try to avoid sugar and refined carbohydrates and eat plenty of fresh, organic vegetables and moderate amounts of whole, fresh fruit.

If you are oestrogen dominant try using natural bio-identical progesterone cream to balance your hormones.

Depression

If you are suffering from long periods of sadness, have lost interest in your favourite activities, and feel worthless, you may have depression. Mood swings are one thing but depression is far more serious. If you have tried, but just can't get yourself feeling positive about life, it may be a good idea to have a chat with your doctor. Depression is an illness and it can be triggered by the chemicals in your brain. Serotonin is the hormone that is responsible for regulating your moods, and when serotonin levels drop due to fluctuating hormones you can experience extreme episodes of depression.

As mentioned before, zinc and copper play an important role in our mental stability, they act as cofactors for enzymes. They are particularly involved in enzymes within brain cells, some of which create the neurotransmitters brain cells use to transmit their messages from one cell to another. The balance of zinc and copper is very important in the brain's regulation of mood. Vitamin B6 is the vitamin most commonly needed by these enzymes, which is why it is often effective in treating depression.

Oestrogen does have positive effects on the brain when it is in balance, but when it is in excess or not balanced by progesterone it can have opposite effects. Help is available and it is important to get the right medication. Natural bio-identical progesterone, anti-depressants and hormone therapy can help. So make an appointment with you doctor to get some more advice. You don't have to feel like this.

Natural Remedies

Sleep - I know this is easier said than done but it can make a difference to your mood swings. Try taking a warm bath before bed and add a few drops of relaxing essential oils such as lavender or chamomile.

Spray – lavender water onto your pillow.

Hops - have a sedative action, though they can be quite bitter to drink, so try mixing them with some lavender and placing by your bedside.

Practice - meditation.

Relax - light a fragranced candle and read a book.

Exercise - to improve your mood.

Eat - a good well balanced diet including B vitamins, cheese, fish, Brazil nuts and whole grains.

Pamper - yourself, buy those new shoes or have a massage.

Have - lunch with friends.

Some - mood enhancing supplements may help, like evening primrose oil, St Johns Wort and ginkgo biloba.

Natural bio-identical progesterone cream to balance oestrogen levels.

Phytomone Spa Therapy - Hormone balancing bath crystals can help bring about a sense of well-being.

Sleep Problems

As we age we do require less sleep, but it seems to be in menopause that we begin losing sleep. Night sweats will obviously be one reason for disturbed sleep and may cause you to waken several times during the night, after which you will probably have difficulty getting back to sleep. Some women experience restless legs, which is another annoying disorder that may keep you awake; this is when you have the urge to move your legs, and is sometimes accompanied by uncomfortable sensations such as throbbing or pulling. Restless legs normally strikes at night or during prolonged periods of sitting or inactivity. Walking around or moving your legs while sitting in bed will help alleviate those unpleasant feelings. There is no known cause, but it has been connected to low iron levels and dopamine abnormalities. Dopamine is a chemical found in the brain and controls muscle activity.

Constant interruptions in your sleep pattern will have a noticeable effect on your daily life and can cause depression, fatigue, increased irritability, tendency towards weight gain, effects on memory and an inability to concentrate on daily tasks.

So for the sake of your sanity it is important to try and find a solution to your sleeping problems.

Cause: Once again our hormones take centre stage here. Fluctuating levels of oestrogen and progesterone can cause sleep disorders, although each one in a different way. The decline of oestrogen slows down the intake of magnesium, a mineral that amongst other things helps our muscles to relax, and oestrogen, as we know, contributes to our hot flushes and night sweats, which can disturb our sleep. Progesterone has a sleep inducing effect, and when levels fall the ability to fall asleep does too. You may also be experiencing psychological problems which are affecting your ability to sleep, such as anxiety, depression, work-related problems or financial issues.

Cure: Try to avoid stimulants before bedtime, such as caffeine and alcohol, and don't exercise late at night. Also try to avoid napping during the day. Take warm baths at bedtime, listen to relaxing music or sounds of nature such as bird songs, tropical rain forest, or flowing water, practice stress relief techniques such as yoga or meditation, and make sure your bedroom is not too hot.
Try as many of the natural remedies as you can, but if you find they are not helping, you may want to try sleeping aids. Discuss it with your doctor to find the best solution for you. He may even suggest a low dose of hormone treatment to bring back restful sleep.
Sleeping pills won't cure your problem and they may make you feel groggy the next morning; you may also become dependent on them, having to increase the dose to maintain the same effect as time goes by, and you may suffer from withdrawal symptoms when you stop taking them. Think carefully before using sleeping pills and use them as a last resort. Make a note on your calendar when you have disturbed sleep so you can check if there is any reoccurring pattern.

Natural Remedies

Chamomile - has a sedative effect. Use it in your evening tea; add one or two teaspoons of the flowers to boiling water and leave to steep for five to ten minutes.
Hops - can be used to make sleep pillows and be kept by your bedside.
Lavender - is one of the most calming herbs and can be used in a

variety of ways to help induce sleep. Use flowers and essential oils in baths, room sprays, sleep sprays, pot-pourri and sleep pillows.

Lemon Balm - is a sedative and stomach soother. Add two to three teaspoons of the dried herb to a cup of boiling water and let it steep for five to ten minutes for a soothing cup of tea that tastes nice too.

Valerian - will help you get off to sleep and reduce night time waking. Use one to two teaspoons of dried valerian root in hot water for a bedtime drink. Take no more than one cup a day as too much can cause headaches.

St. Johns Wort - will help relieve insomnia and mild depression due to an imbalance in brain chemistry. Most commonly taken in capsule form. St. Johns Wort should not be taken with certain other medications such as prescribed anti-depressants or the contraceptive pill, so check to see if it is compatible with any other medications you are taking.

Read - to relax, but choose your reading material with care. You don't want to stimulate your mind too much, so keep reports and manuals out of the way and choose something enjoyable and light.

Listen to soft music which can have calming effects, or alternatively, listening to nature sounds can be very relaxing.

Meditation or prayer may help you relax and be at peace with whatever is on your mind.

A warm bath may make you drowsy and ready for bed; make it as relaxing as possible by dimming the lights or using candles, burn lavender oil and add two cups of the **Phytomone Spa Therapy bath crystals** to your bath water. This can ease sore muscles and balance your hormones with the carefully blended herbs specifically chosen for menopausal symptoms. Take a few deep breaths and relax.

Stretching helps the body to relax tense muscles and bring warmth to the joints and surrounding tissues. Lie on your bed and stretch your arms and legs and feel the energy move through your body.

Try and keep your room dark, light suppresses the sleep hormone melatonin, so darkness will help you stay asleep. The pineal gland is an important brain regulator and is very sensitive to light, so by keeping your room dark your pineal gland tells your brain it's night time and time to sleep.

Invest in blinds or black out curtains to block out any external lighting, such as street lamps or security lighting - or buy a sleep mask.

Make sure your room is cool. It's better to sleep in a cooler room than an overheated one. The ideal temperature for sleeping is 65 degrees and 65 percent humidity.

Change your bed linens weekly and enjoy the feel of the clean, crisp fresh smelling sheets.

Spritz your pillow and room with lavender water.

Natural bio-identical progesterone cream to balance oestrogen levels

Memory and Concentration Problems

Our memory starts to decline from around the age of 20. So by the time we reach the grand old age of menopause you would think we would have adjusted to short term memory loss and fuzzy thinking. Still it seems to come out of nowhere and these 'senior moments' can be very frustrating when we have lost our glasses for the tenth time that day, can't remember where the car keys are, have a tendency to repeat ourselves and seem to have acquired the inability to focus and concentrate on everyday tasks as our mind wanders off.

Cause: Declining oestrogen levels have a strong effect on the functions of the brain including verbal word fluency (the ability to remember names and words), language skills and moods. This decline also has an effect on our neurotransmitters in the brain (acetylcholine, serotonin and norepinephrine) which regulate cognitive functions, including memory and the ability to concentrate. Other factors affecting you may include lack of sleep, poor diet and vitamin deficiencies, some medications including sleeping pills and anti-depressants, excess amounts of alcohol and of course natural ageing.

Cure: Exercise will improve your circulation, helping your blood carry more oxygen and energy to your brain, making you more alert and able to concentrate. You can also try some of the brain exercises we have included in this book to help keep your brain active. Meditate to practice your concentration skills and to also calm your overloaded mind – and of course a good night's sleep will always help.

Natural Remedies

Brain exercises - for mental stimulation, focus and concentration.

Meditation - to control you mind and promote calmness.

Exercise - to improve oxygen supply to your brain, making you more alert.

Improved Diet - include more oily fish and eggs.

Ginseng - to improve memory function.

Ginkgo Biloba - to improve blood circulation and oxygen flow to the body and brain.

Sleep - to re-energise your brain.

Fish Oil supplements - for omega 3.

Rosemary - to keep the brain stimulated.

Green Tea - or black tea to promote healthy blood flow.

Fatigue

Apart from hot flushes, fatigue is one of the most frequently experienced symptoms of menopause, which is hardly surprising if your sleep is being constantly disturbed by night sweats, restless legs and sleep disorders. Even if you do manage to sleep, fatigue can affect you, as it involves lack of energy rather than drowsiness.

Cause: As our oestrogen and progesterone levels drop so do our energy levels. Other common conditions for fatigue could be thyroid disorder, adrenal fatigue or depression.

Cure: Begin by making a few lifestyle changes. Nutrition is very important and you should be eating 'energy type foods' to help raise blood glucose levels. The best way of doing this is to eat 'good carbs', the ones that will produce a gradual and sustained release of energy. Avoid refined carbs that will give you a quick sugar rush; they may give you that quick energy high but they will also drop you back down quickly as well. You need to take an interest in your nutrition and make sure you eat sensibly and well. If your body has all the nutrition it needs, it will serve you well and help you cope with stress, illness and fatigue. Fatigue is one more reason for you to exercise. Keeping active gives you more energy, so break through the vicious circle of - no energy, no exercise and work through your fatigue. After a couple of days your energy levels will rise and so will your mood.

If you haven't been exercising for a while and the thought of exercise makes your blood run cold, then start off by going for a brisk 10 minute walk to get your body moving and circulation flowing, and maybe look for yoga or tai chi classes in your area, which is a gentler form of exercise but very effective.

Skin brushing is also great for improving circulation and to give you that 'awake' feeling.

Take the time to look after yourself and do something self-indulgent on a regular basis; it doesn't always have to involve money, just something you enjoy, maybe an art exhibition, gallery opening, anything that interests you and makes you feel good, because if you feel good about yourself then your whole attitude towards your problems will change – you will feel more positive about solving them instead of allowing them to overtake your life. Have some fun and if you don't already put any effort into socialising then start now. Invite friends over for supper or organise some social event. Someone has to do it and most people are happy to rely on others to sort it out – so get organised and have some fun.

Feng Shui experts believe that clutter saps your energy, so why not clear out. Start with your bedroom and turn it into a peaceful haven for you to sleep. De-clutter, organise your clothes, hang things up, throw things away, clean the windows, dust, vacuum, change the bed linens, empty bins, put magazines and papers away and make it all clean and sparkly. Finish off with some pot-pourri, essential oils or room fragrance to create a calming, relaxing atmosphere. This new haven may also help with your sleeping disorder.

Now you just have the rest of the house to do!

Natural Remedies

Revised diet - eat plenty of the good carbs and unprocessed natural foods such as whole grains, fruits, vegetables, lean meats and other protein sources. Avoid over-consumption of dairy and over-processed foods. Raw seeds and nuts, except peanuts, are a good source of essential fatty acids. A healthy diet helps your liver process toxins far more efficiently, the fewer toxins you have in your body the more energised you will feel.

Drink - dandelion tea and milk thistle to cleanse the liver.

Seaweeds - of all kinds help nourish the nervous, immune and hormonal systems.

Ginseng - will improve vitality.

Ginger - will help boost your circulation. Try putting fresh ginger in a cup of hot water.

Liquorice - is immune enhancing and boosts adrenal functions.

Gotu Kola - improves brain function memory, anti-stress, anti-anxiety, and is a relaxant.

St Johns Wort - helps relieve depression that is a cause or effect of fatigue.

Yerba Mate - stimulates like caffeine but without the nervousness. Calming, anti-oxidant and increases oxygen to the heart and brain.

Exercise - the more you do the more energised you will feel; work through the fatigue barrier and get moving.

Indulge yourself - you don't need a reason or an excuse, life is too short .

Socialise - and have fun.

De-Clutter - and clean your space.

Meditate for a calm mind.

Try - tai chi or yoga.

Phytomone Spa Therapy body oil to nourish the skin and bring about a sense of well-being.

Anxiety

Can put you on the edge, making you feel that a disaster is just around the corner. You worry about every day events and always expect the worst to happen. Anxiety can also lead to heart palpitations, fatigue, shortness of breath, digestive problems, muscle aches and panic attacks, where you experience acute episodes of overwhelming fear or panic.

Cause: Oestrogen and progesterone levels have a significant effect on the brain's regulation of moods and emotions. If you are not normally prone to anxiety you will probably find these symptoms subside when your hormones are in balance.

Cure: Try some of the natural remedies suggested for fatigue. If they become too severe and you feel unable to cope, then you must discuss it with you doctor to find alternative treatment.

Dizziness

Many women report bouts of dizziness during menopause, with sensations of light-headedness and imbalance, possibly accompanied by nausea.

Cause: Changes in hormone levels can produce changes in the blood vessels, causing your brain to receive an inadequate supply of blood. Other causes for dizziness may include low blood sugar (hypoglycaemia), low blood pressure and dehydration.
If your dizzy spells are severe and become more frequent you should consult your doctor, especially if you experience trouble breathing, chest pains, change in speech or vision and loss of consciousness. In very rare cases dizziness during menopause can indicate a more serious condition.

Cure: Treatment for dizziness should begin with lifestyle changes, eat healthy, get enough fluids and exercise. If you are prone to dizziness make sure to take care when standing up too quickly or making any sudden postural changes.

Natural Remedies
Eat - complex carbs to keep blood sugar stable.
Black tea - crushed ginger or ginger root capsules will help with nausea.
Make - sure you have enough iron and folic acid in your diet, it is available in foods such as fish, poultry, lean meats, and green leafy vegetables.
Vitamin B12 - is necessary for proper red blood cell formation and is found in fish, meat, poultry, eggs and milk products. This vitamin is not generally present in plant foods.
Exercise - to improve circulation and to ensure your brain is receiving enough blood.

Headache and Migraines
Some women will experience an influx of headaches when they enter peri-menopause. There are several types of headaches you may get, ranging from a mild to severe migraine, and with symptoms such as a throbbing pain in the head, intense pain in a specific area, nausea, sensitivity to noise and light and pain lasting up to twenty four hours or longer. Tension headaches are the most common, with the feeling of a tight band being pressed around your head, which can also cause tension and pain in the back of your neck at the base of your skull.

Cause: Fluctuating hormones. Oestrogen causes blood vessels to dilate, while progesterone causes them to constrict. As the hormones fluctuate the blood vessels are forced to expand and contract, resulting in head pain. If you suffered from headaches during your menstrual periods you will probably suffer during menopause and they may be even more severe.

Cure: A good diet will help level out hormone imbalances to a certain degree, which may help alleviate the problem, and non-prescription drugs such as aspirin or ibuprofen can offer relief. Progesterone can help promote normal vascular tone and help prevent headaches or migraines. Using natural bio-identical progesterone cream may help to balance your hormones.
Try and keep a note on your calendar to see if there is anything specific that triggers your headaches or migraines. If a pattern does show up it will make it easier for you to eliminate whatever is causing the problem.

Natural Remedies
Drink - a large glass of water, dehydration can cause headaches.
Massage - head and skull to relieve tension.
Aromatherapy - used in diffusers, candles and burning oils, Sandalwood, peppermint, eucalyptus, lavender and chamomile can all help soothe headaches.
Ice Packs - may help. Apply to pained area for 10 to 15 minutes.
Phytomone Spa Therapy Cooling gel helps when applied to temples and along hair line.
Hot shower - cascading hot water, down your neck and back may help alleviate pain.
Diet - identification of any trigger points - chocolate, dairy products, wheat and eggs are quite common triggers.
Calcium - and magnesium can help muscles relax and increase blood flow; dolomite supplements - a combination of calcium and magnesium may help.
Natural Bio-identical progesterone cream to balance hormones.

Joint Pain
Joint pain, also known as 'arthralgia' is defined by stiffness or swelling in or around the joint. The pain often occurs in high impact

joints such as knees, hips and back. You may also experience pain in the joints in your hands. Typical joint discomfort related to menopause includes pain, stiffness and swelling.

Cause: Oestrogen affects joints by keeping inflammation down. Inflammation is the main cause of joint pain. As our oestrogen levels diminish during peri-menopause our joints get less and less oestrogen and pain is often the result.

Cure: Physical activity such as walking or simple stretching and some muscle- strengthening exercises may all help to alleviate joint pain. If you find exercise too painful, try doing it in water. Consult your doctor before starting any new exercise routine if you have severe joint problems. Revise your diet - inflammation can be caused by a diet that's too high in refined carbohydrates and sugars and too low in essential fatty acids. Alternative medicine and acupuncture may also offer some relief.

Natural Remedies
Warm Baths - are highly beneficial, add **Phytomone Spa Therapy** bath crystals to help relax the muscles.
Massage - with warm oil - try eucalyptus and menthol.
Drink - papaya seed tea to provide some relief.
Turmeric powder - dissolve ½ teaspoon of turmeric powder in warm water three times a day.
Carrot juice - will help strengthen ligaments.
Apple cider vinegar - added to a warm glass of water - two teaspoons - add honey to taste if required.
Alternate - hot and cold compresses on painful areas.
Increase - intake of omega 3 oils.
Exercise - to increase joint flexibility and strengthen bones; exercise in water if it's too painful.

Quick Exercises For Joint Flexibility
To help alleviate stiffness try these simple exercises at home as and when needed.

Toes – Sit on floor, legs straight out in front of you, flex toes 10 times.

Ankles – Rotate in each direction 10 times while sitting.
Knees – Bend, lift, and straighten, 10 times each leg.
Hips – Bend left leg, left foot on right thigh, hold left knee with left hand and left ankle with right hand, gently bounce knee up and down, change sides and repeat.
Fingers – Arms out shoulder height, keep straight and stretch out fingers and then close over thumbs, repeat 10 times.
Wrists – Arms out straight, rotate wrists clockwise 10 times, anti-clockwise 10 times.
Elbows Arms out, palms up, bend at elbows, touch shoulders with fingers, straighten out again, repeat 10 times.
Shoulders – Arms bent, fingers touching shoulders, make circular movements with elbows clockwise 10 times, anticlockwise 10 times.
Spine – Sit on floor, legs straight out in front of you, reach forward and touch legs without bending knees, repeat 20 times.
Waist – Stand up and slowly reach down to touch toes, bending from waist, try to keep knees straight, repeat 10 times – Remain standing, feet two feet apart, side bends, arms over head, repeat five times each side.

Muscle Tension

You may be affected by muscle tension during menopause, where your muscles feel taught and strained especially in the back, shoulders and neck. It may also be accompanied by tension headaches, stress and anxiety, fatigue and muscle spasms.

Cause: When our oestrogen levels drop it causes the stress hormone cortisol to rise. This imbalance of hormones raises our blood pressure and blood sugar, and the muscles in the body tighten and become fatigued.
Excess copper can also cause muscle pain. This can be a result of being oestrogen dominate – try using natural bio-identical progesterone cream to balance this effect.

Cure: You need to adapt a healthy lifestyle which includes good nutrition and exercise. Some muscles respond well to warmth, so massages, warm baths and showers will help ease the pain.
Phytomone Spa Therapy Bath Crystals will help muscle tension; add a cup full to your bath water. If your muscle pain is severe and

affecting your daily life, you may require a stronger form of medication from your doctor to help ease the pain.

Natural Remedies
Warm baths - and showers.
Massage - using the hormone balancing oil from the **Phytomone Spa Therapy** range.
Exercise - try swimming.
Breathing exercises.
Relax - listen to music, light candles and burn incense.
Use - natural progesterone cream to bring about hormonal balance.

Skin Changes
Most women notice a change in their skin during and after menopause and complain mainly of loss of firmness, elasticity and dryness. Unfortunately, there is no stopping the ageing process. From the moment we are born we start to age and by the time we have spent forty-plus years on planet Earth, gravity, sun damage and a host of other things all start to take their toll.

Cause: Oestrogen is very involved in the normal function of the skin, and the diminished levels during the menopause transition will contribute to a decline in elastin and collagen fibres, which support the skin, giving it firmness and smoothness. Lack of oestrogen decreases the blood vessel supply to the skin; the sebaceous glands shrink and produce less oil, resulting in dryer skin. The deeper fat layers become thinner and as skin thins it becomes pale and translucent, making it more susceptible to developing thread veins and broken capillaries. Another common symptom you may experience is itchy skin, which can feel like a tingly sensation or a feeling of something crawling in or under the skin; a symptom known as formication. This happens because the skin becomes hypersensitive due to the thinning of both the surface and underlying muscles that support it. Your skin will now also become more sensitive to sunburn, windy and dry conditions and possibly allergens. Remember the sun is the number one ageing factor; the sun's rays damage our DNA and diminish the capability for genes and cells to communicate properly to fight the ageing process, causing the skin to sag and lose its elasticity. Make sure your day creams and body lotions contain an SPF of at least 15.

The decline in collagen is greatest in the years just after menopause – about 30 percent of skin collagen is lost during the first five years after menopause and about two percent every year after that.

Cure: Unfortunately, we can't turn back the clock, but we can take preventative measures to delay the ageing process for as long as possible, and that means starting from the inside and working out. Your diet should include all the vitamins and minerals your skin needs - zinc and copper keep the skin supple and can be found in yoghurt, turkey, sesame seeds, sunflower seeds, soybeans and barley. Vitamin C and E have important anti-oxidants and protect the skin from free radicals. Fruits and vegetables are all good sources of vitamins and minerals and should be included in your daily diet. Fibre is important to prevent constipation, which can affect the appearance of the skin, and try to include more fish in your diet to boost omega 3 levels.
More detailed information on skin care and products is available in the Body and Soul chapter.

Natural Remedies
Wear - a sunscreen.
Eat - a healthy diet.
Drink - plenty of water to stay hydrated.
Practice - the facial exercises we have included.
Exfoliate - regularly.
Keep skin well moisturised with the **Phytomone** range of products specifically designed for hormonally changing skin.
Facials - and massages help circulation.

Hair Changes
It is normal to lose about 50 to 100 hairs each day, they are constantly regenerated by your hair follicles. However, if you find you are losing a lot more hair than normal, or you notice clumps of hair coming out when you wash and brush it, then you are probably one of the 50 percent of women who suffer from hair loss and thinning during menopause.

Cause: The two main hormones involved here are oestrogen and testosterone. The imbalance causes the hair follicles to shrink, pushing hairs out sooner than is normal.

Testosterone is also responsible for hirsutism, which is the presence of excess hair. You may find hairs growing on your chin, upper lip, cheeks, and chest, and they are normally coarser than the hair on your head.

Thinning hair is often genetic, so if your parents suffered from it, it's most likely you will too.

Cure: A change in diet may help slightly - try increasing your intake of protein, vitamins B & C and iron. Exercise will improve circulation and techniques such as yoga or meditation will reduce stress. Specialist shampoos are available from chemists, which help promote hair growth. If you find yourself with a few hairs sprouting on your face, the simplest solution is to pull them out with tweezers; alternatively you could try electrolysis for a more permanent result. More information on this is available in the Body and Soul Chapter.

Natural Remedies
Improve diet
Exercise
Use specialist shampoos

Tender Breasts

Most women will have experienced tender breasts, normally a few days before their period starts, and for some it can be uncomfortable, but there is usually no cause for concern.

Cause: The most common cause of sore breasts during menopause is due to hormonal changes. We know oestrogen levels drop during menopause, but you could still be oestrogen dominant if your progesterone levels have dropped too. This can cause glandular tissues to increase, causing the fibrous tissues to stretch and become painful; it may also be accompanied by fluid retention. Once your hormone levels begin to level out the symptoms should subside.

Cure: Vitamins E and B6 will help with the soreness - try to include extra amounts in your diet - calcium can also be beneficial. You may be lacking in essential fatty acids, so try taking a supplement of evening primrose oil and eat more omega 3 fatty acids found in fish and flaxseeds, and discuss with your doctor the use of a natural bio-identical progesterone cream. Buy a good bra, make sure you get the right size, and wear a special sport's bra when exercising.

Natural Remedies
Increase - intake of calcium, B6, Vitamin E and essential fatty acids.
Avoid caffeine.
Buy - a good bra.
Relax - in a warm bath.
Natural Bio-Identical Progesterone Cream.

Urinary Tract Problems
Frequent urination
Incontinence
Painful urination
When oestrogen levels fall the muscles weaken, including the bladder muscle, which can cause frequent urination and slight urine leakage when coughing, laughing, sneezing or maybe lifting something heavy. Painful urination indicates an infection and you will need a course of antibiotics to clear it up. Infections may occur due to the thinning of the lining of the urethra and bladder.

Cause: Mainly due to weakened bladder muscles caused by lack of oestrogen, though progesterone also plays an important role in preventing vaginal and urinary tract infections. Oestrogen and progesterone help each other; oestrogen is necessary for cells to make progesterone receptors, and progesterone helps make oestrogen receptors more sensitive. When progesterone is deficient, oestrogen receptors become less sensitive to oestrogen, causing women to have signs of oestrogen deficiency, even though this is not the case. When progesterone is restored to normal physiological levels, oestrogen receptors become more sensitive and signs of oestrogen deficiency disappear. Progesterone is also part of our immune defence system that prevents infections.

Cure: Pelvic floor exercises will help strengthen the bladder muscles and you will be able to regain some control. If you have a bladder infection avoid products that are perfumed in your personal hygiene routine, wear cotton underwear to minimise moisture retention, and drink unsweetened cranberry juice to maintain the PH balance of your urine. For more severe cases consult your doctor who will advise you on the best course of treatment.

Natural Remedies
Pelvic floor exercises.
Wear - underwear.
Drink –cranberry juice.
Drink spinach juice or coconut water (nitrates and potassium make this effective).

Vaginal Dryness
During the menopausal transition 40 to 60 percent of women will experience some sort of problem involving vaginal dryness. Normally the body naturally lubricates the vaginal walls with a thin layer of moisture, which is excreted through the blood vessel walls around the vagina. When a woman becomes aroused these blood vessels receive more blood flow, which stimulates the fluids and increases vaginal lubrication. Lack of lubrication can cause discomfort, especially during intercourse, and can affect your sexual desire and pleasure. Other symptoms may include stinging, burning, irritation, urinary frequency and general discomfort. Itching is normally an indication of an infection and you may need a course of antibiotics to clear it up.

Cause: Reduced oestrogen levels cause the walls of the vagina to become thinner, dryer and less elastic; vaginal secretion also diminishes, causing a decrease in lubrication. In addition low oestrogen changes the PH level of the vagina, making the once acidic environment more alkaline, which can increase irritation and the likelihood of vaginal infection.

Cure: Foods containing phyto-oestrogens such as flaxseeds and dark green leafy vegetables will produce a mild oestrogen like effect and may help in increasing moisture in the vagina. Try sprinkling ground flaxseed on your cereals, salads, pastas, and include more fresh vegetables whenever possible. Vaginal lubricants can offer some relief, such as KY Jelly or Aloe Vera. Vaginal moisturisers like Replens or one containing a low dose of oestrogen may help alleviate dryness. Each cream will be slightly different so you might need to experiment with a few to find the right one. Alternatively, oral hormone therapy may be a better option for you and you should discuss this with your doctor.

Natural Remedies
Lubricating creams.
Black Cohosh
Diet - rich in phyto-oestrogens, B Vitamins and Vitamin E.
Topical creams - containing liquorice have proven effective.
Sesame oil - try massaging the walls of your vagina with this oil.
Aloe Vera - juice known for its moisturising properties; try mixing with almond milk or soymilk and drink.
Pelvic floor - exercises to increase muscle strength, increase circulation and boost vaginal moisture levels.
Avoid - highly perfumed bath products, soaps, bath oils and bubble baths which can all promote dryness.
Antihistamines - often taken for allergies, dry out mucous membranes, including vaginal tissues.

Loss of Libido
The term 'libido' has long been used to describe a person's sexual desire. Loss of libido or desire for sex may have its roots in hormone imbalance, but psychological and physical factors also play a part. Low self-esteem, poor body image, vaginal dryness and irritation, feeling exhausted, headaches...........no wonder you don't feel sexy – what is a woman to do?

Cause: First let's look at how your hormonal imbalance is affecting you. The three major hormones that contribute to the reduction of sexual drive and desire are:
Oestrogen - low levels of oestrogen will cause changes in the vulva and vagina as the blood supply diminishes, the vulva area becomes paler, thinner and less plump and there is a gradual loss of pubic hair. Lack of oestrogen is also the cause of vaginal dryness, lack of blood supply causes a decrease in lubrication.
Progesterone - can cause loss of libido due to the low levels. Remember that oestrogen production falls only 40 to 60 percent at menopause, whereas progesterone which is normally at its highest at

ovulation, and when a woman is most fertile, falls to almost zero when ovulation no longer occurs - so it makes sense that a lack of progesterone may have some effect on our libido.

Testosterone - women make about a tenth as much testosterone as men, which gradually declines with age. Testosterone levels of a peri-menopausal woman tend to be about half that of a woman in her early twenties and the steepest decline is around the time of menopause, resulting in a falling libido. Testosterone can be prescribed to women to help improve sex drive. If you think this may help you, then have a chat with your doctor and he will advise the best type of treatment. Make sure you weigh up all the pros and cons before you begin any treatment, because although testosterone replacement may increase your sexual interest, the down side is it may also increase your cholesterol levels, cause excessive facial and body hair and weight gain.

Apart from your hormone imbalance, there may be other issues that are affecting your sexual desire. If you are used to a fairly active sex life and it has dwindled down to once a week, once a month or less than that, it could begin to affect both you and your partner. The last thing you need in your life right now is more stress and misunderstanding.

Regardless of how many times you have sex or don't have it, if it's affecting your relationship then it can become a problem.

You need to explain to your partner what's happening to you and why. Chances are he will have no idea how you are feeling, or what's actually happening to you, both mentally and physically; he is probably thinking you don't find him attractive anymore and is feeling hurt and rejected. Communication is the key. Tell him how you are feeling about your body, your insecurities, and how it is uncomfortable to have sex because of the dryness. Then explain in a very simplified form, because that is all he will really want to know, about your hormone imbalance, what it means and how it is affecting you. Once he has been reassured that it is nothing to do with him, you will be able to work together to find new solutions to improving your sex life.

Now, what about you? What can you do to get your mojo back and start feeling sexy again?

Well, your mental attitude towards menopause might be quite relevant here. Back in the day when women didn't really live much beyond menopause, it was thought that you were coming towards the end of your life, so there was no desire to have any sort of positive attitude towards life after menopause. However, as we know in today's world, women can live well into their eighties, and should be capable of enjoying an active sex life for a while to come.

This second stage of your life really should be all about you. Time has given you experience, wisdom and confidence, so don't let a few pesky little hormones or misunderstandings stand in the way of enjoying life.

As you develop this new relationship with yourself, you will have to adjust your routine and take certain things into account, but this could be a blessing in disguise. You are almost forced into changing your habits, and what you have been doing for the last decade or so of your life - now needs to change. This can be inspiring and uplifting, giving you the motivation you need to see things in a new light. If you are feeling good about yourself, it will affect how you respond to all daily situations and not just your sex life.

If you exercise and follow a good diet, you know you are doing your very best to look after your body. It will repay you by looking good. You will have more energy, and hopefully a lot of the other menopausal symptoms will become less severe.

By middle age most couples have developed a routine for sex – same time, same place and even the same day of the week, so this could be a good opportunity to discuss and strengthen your current relationship - or maybe reconsider a bad one!

Variety can be the spice in your sex life, and if you have a strong, secure relationship now could be the perfect time to try something different and put the sizzle back into it.Don't forget that your partner may also be dealing with his own sexual issues. It is quite common from around the age of 40 for men to have problems with their erections, and they may need more stimulation. Once again, your menopause could be a blessing in disguise, giving you the opportunity to communicate with each other and strengthen your relationship.

Cure: A low dose of natural testosterone, along with natural bio-identical progesterone cream may be a benefit to you and help restore your libido. Do bear in mind you are trying to balance your hormones, so it is important to get the correct dosage. You want the equivalent to normal body function - more is not better. If you exceed the dose it could inhibit your sex drive. Exercise, not only for the obvious health benefits, but to help you feel good about your image, knowing that you are the best that you can be, is a great self-image boost. You may even surprise yourself at how wonderful you are. Make sure your diet contains all the right nutrients for optimum health (more of this in the diet and nutrition chapter), and also include lean red meats, liver, oysters for zinc, leafy greens and almonds for magnesium, and fish and nuts for protein.

Pelvic floor exercises will help strengthen your muscles.

A mutual understanding with your partner will help strengthen your relationship and improve your sex life.

Explore your senses, try something different or organise a spontaneous weekend away and fall in love with your partner all over again.

Natural Remedies
Romantic baths.
Sensual massage.
Sensual lotions and potions.
Tantric sex.

See the Body and Soul Chapter for more help and ideas.

Bone Health and Calcium Requirements

Our bones are made up of collagen (protein), calcium salts and other minerals. Each bone has a thick outer shell and a strong inner mesh of bone, which looks a little like a honeycomb.

Most people think of their bones as rigid structures, but they are alive and constantly changing and regenerating throughout your life. Old worn bone is broken down by cells called 'osteoclasts' and replaced by bone building cells called 'osteoblasts'.

In childhood osteoblasts work faster, enabling the skeleton to increase in density and strength. During this period of rapid bone growth, it takes the skeleton just two years to completely renew itself. In adults the process takes seven to ten years.

Without adequate levels of oestrogen and progesterone, bones aren't able to absorb the proper amounts of calcium to replenish bone mass as cells die off. The body also has trouble controlling the amount of bone cells that are destroyed without oestrogen to regulate the function. Oestrogens most important effect on bone health is osteoporosis, where it appears to be the prevention of bone breakdown, known as 're-sorption'. Healthy bones require a balance of osteoclasts and osteoblasts. As oestrogen levels diminish, the osteoclasts (responsible for the breakdown of bone) seem to live longer than the osteoblasts; this leads to bones being broken down at a rate much greater than they can be rebuilt, causing them to grow weak and brittle. This may be brought about by a lack of progesterone. Where oestrogen's job is to slow down bone loss, progesterone plays the lead role in building bone.

Exercise is a great way to stimulate your bones to become stronger and help slow the process of decline to prevent fractures and osteoporosis. The two most important kinds of exercise to strengthen bones are:

Weight bearing aerobic exercises

Weight lifting/muscle strengthening exercises

Weight bearing exercises use bone and muscle to work against gravity. Working against resistance will increase bone density. Include exercises such as stair climbing, brisk walking, jogging, tai chi, yoga, Pilates and dancing.

Weight lifting/muscle strengthening exercises will improve your muscle mass and bone strength. Weights will overload your muscles, which will respond by getting stronger, the pull on the muscle on the bone has a similar effect of strengthening the bone. Use hand weights, dumbbells and ankle weights when working out. Squats are good for building bone density in your legs, pelvis and back and can also be performed holding dumbbells. If you find them particularly challenging, try doing them against a wall for some support. Forearm curls with weights will improve arm strength.

If you have been diagnosed with osteoporosis you may need to be careful of vigorous exercise and avoid movements that bend, twist and flex the spine too much, but it is important to stay active and to find something that you enjoy such as walking, golf, gardening or tai chi. Swimming is also a good all round exercise that doesn't stress our bones too much.

Teeth

Let's not forget that our teeth are bones too and can suffer from the same effects as the rest of your bones during menopause.

Pay attention to your dental hygiene, brush your teeth at least twice a day, and especially after meals if possible. If your teeth have become sensitive due to thinning of enamel, use toothpaste formulated for sensitive teeth. Avoid using a toothbrush with hard bristles as it may irritate or damage the gums, and don't forget to clean between your teeth by flossing or using a brush designed for this. Finish off by using a mouthwash to help remove any remaining bacteria.

Visit your dentist for regular check-ups and to have your teeth cleaned and polished.

Calcium

98 to 99 percent of our calcium is stored in our bones and if you don't get enough from your daily diet your body will start to steal it from your bones - long term this can lead to fragile bones and osteoporosis.

Calcium is absorbed in our intestines and the kidneys eliminate any excess amounts. In addition to strengthening the bones, calcium is extremely important for the contraction of muscles, including the heart muscle. Low or high levels of calcium can quickly lead to disturbances in the cardiac rhythm.

After menopause, calcium is lost from the bones at a greater rate, and in addition to this, since oestrogen assists in the absorption of calcium from food, once the oestrogen levels fall the body becomes less efficient at absorbing calcium. The body's natural ability to absorb calcium decreases with age, it can only be absorbed in small doses at a time. Spread out your intake throughout the day to 500mg at a time. If you think you may not be getting enough calcium try keeping a calcium diary for a week or two to see how much you are getting – you might be surprised to learn that your diet is providing you with adequate amounts of calcium, which isn't that difficult to achieve. Remember that the source of all calcium is from the soil or the sea in the form of shells and coral. Calcium is technically a metal found mostly in rocks. Soils containing those rocks absorb calcium from them, which is in turn absorbed by the plants grown in that soil. When animals or humans then eat those plants, they ingest the calcium they contain. As the cycle continues, when humans eat or drink the products from those animals, we then receive the calcium from there as well. Our best edible source of calcium is from plants - not, as you may think, from cow's milk, as the dairy companies would have us believe. Even cows get their calcium from plant sources, along with added undesirable growth hormones which are passed on to us! A simple rule to remember - all dark green leafy vegetables are a good source of calcium, and should be eaten often, with the exception of spinach, which blocks calcium absorption. If you are falling short of the recommended daily allowance of 1500mg for whatever reason, you may want to consider taking a calcium supplement. However, you will need correct amounts of magnesium for calcium to be absorbed efficiently. Calcium supplements are available as either - calcium carbonate, which comes from rocks, mainly limestone, and oyster shells - or calcium citrate, which is the calcium salt of citric acid. Calcium carbonate tends to be more common because it's cheap and readily available. However, calcium citrate is better absorbed by the body. When taking calcium carbonate supplements you will need to take them with food to help with the absorption, whereas calcium citrate can be taken on an empty stomach. Bear in mind that both types of supplements will not be one hundred percent calcium. Check the label for the percentage, usually calcium carbonate is about 40 percent calcium and calcium citrate contains about 21 percent, but as mentioned it is better absorbed. Alternatively, you could use a Dolomite supplement, which is a combination of calcium and magnesium.

Foods That Block Calcium Absorption
Sometimes foods that are considered very healthy and nutritious contain calcium that your body can't absorb due to oxalic acid and phytic acid. These substances bind together with the calcium in the food containing it, making it nearly impossible to absorb. These acids don't affect other foods that you are eating during the same meal.

Look out for:

- Spinach
- Soybeans

- Rhubarb
- Cocoa

Even though these foods inhibit calcium absorption, experts agree that the benefits you derive from the other important nutrients, especially spinach, far outweigh the negative effects of their nature to block calcium. Just be aware they won't count towards your daily RDA for calcium.

Calcium Depleters
We know we need calcium in our diet to protect our bones and teeth, but we also need to keep it there. Some foods and drinks can leach calcium from your body.

Caffeine and Sugar
They create an acid environment in the body which is offset by drawing calcium from the bones.

Animal Proteins and Dairy Products
Are also responsible for creating an acidic environment in the body which is corrected by leaching calcium from the bones. Animal and dairy products can increase both calcium intake and calcium excretion and the overall net gain can be low. Plant proteins in beans, grains and vegetables do not appear to have this effect.

Fizzy Drinks
Can contain relatively high levels of phosphorous. In order to balance these levels, calcium is drawn from the bones and teeth. Caffeinated fizzy drinks are particularly harmful.

Alcohol
Can damage osteoblasts (bone building cells) and inhibit absorption of calcium.

Salt
Can cause leaching of calcium from the bones and an excess urinary excretion of calcium.

Smoking
Although not a food, it is worth mentioning that the toxins in cigarettes have a negative effect on the bones and contribute to bone loss.

Vitamins and Mineral Requirements

Calcium RDA = 1500mg
Sources = Fermented soy, almonds, broccoli, kale, watercress sardines and salmon (with bones) sunflower seeds, sesame seeds, oats, dairy products, figs and prunes.

Vitamin D is very important because it is crucial for the proper absorption of calcium. Without this vitamin you are not going to be able to put calcium to as good a use as you need to, especially during menopause.
Vitamin D is a fat-soluble vitamin and is naturally present in very few foods, but it is added to some and is also available as a supplement. The main source of Vitamin D is from the sunlight. When we expose our skin to the UVA rays the body converts it into Vitamin D and stores it in our fat. Most of us will get enough sunlight to help our bones just by being out and about during the day doing our chores –10 to 15 minutes each day is all you need.
RDA = 600 IUs
Sources = Egg yolks, liver, fish oils, kippers, mackerel, oysters, salmon, tuna, dandelion greens, mushrooms, peanuts, raisins, pears, and sunlight.

Magnesium is a mineral and is needed to convert Vitamin D into the actual form that the body can use.
RDA = 400mg
Sources = Salmon, halibut, green leafy vegetables, sesame seeds, flax seeds, apricots, apples, avocados, brown rice, tofu, and whole grains.

Boron is another mineral which is necessary to increase calcium uptake, has mild oestrogen properties, enhances brain function and promotes alertness.
RDA = 3.0mg
Sources = Apples, carrots, grapes, dark green leafy vegetables, raw nuts, pears and whole grains.

Vitamin K helps promote strong bones by binding calcium and other minerals to the bone. This vitamin plays an important role in

the intestines and aids in converting glucose into glycogen.
RDA = 60-65mcg
Sources = Asparagus, broccoli, Brussel sprouts, cabbage,
cauliflower, dark green leafy vegetables, egg yolks, liver, oatmeal
safflower oil, soybeans, yoghurt.

Vitamin B6 supports calcium absorption, metabolises foods into
energy and helps maintain normal homocysteine levels (amino acids
produced by the body, usually as a by-product of consuming meat).
Elevated levels may be associated with atherosclerosis, as well as an
increased risk of heart disease and strokes.
RDA = 1.5mg
Sources = Chicken, turkey, beef, pork, cod, tuna, trout, halibut, bell
peppers, spinach, broccoli, asparagus, sunflower seeds, wholegrains,
soybeans and lentils.

RDA = Recommend daily allowance
IU = International Units
MCG = Micrograms
MG = Milligrams
(1 mcg = 40 IU)

Hormone Replacement Therapy

It is important to remember that your loss of oestrogen and
progesterone is part of the natural ageing process and you don't have
to supplement it to be healthy. However, some women suffer such
serious hormone imbalances that they find it difficult to function on
a daily basis. If you have severe menopause symptoms and a change
in your diet and lifestyle has had little or no effect, then hormone
replacement therapy (HRT) may give you the relief you are looking
for.

The phrase hormone replacement therapy can be slightly misleading,
in as much as it suggests the drug is actually 'replacing' all the
hormones that have been lost, whereas in fact, the dosage is well
below that of what an average premenopausal woman would

normally produce. To avoid any confusion most people now refer to it as Hormone Therapy (HT).

HT was developed in the 1940s as a method of supplementing the oestrogen lost both during and after the menopause and to help alleviate many of the symptoms it brought about, including hot flushes and vaginal dryness; it was also thought to reduce the risk of osteoporosis. However, in the mid-1970's, research confirmed that using oestrogen alone significantly increased the risk of cancer of the uterus , so progestogen; a synthetic version of progesterone, was added to protect the womb. HT was then re-launched and marketed as a 'wonder drug'. But unfortunately its image has never quite recovered and hormone therapy has become recognised as a medication with both positive and negative effects.

The main hormones contained in HT are oestrogen and progestogen, which can be derived from different sources but they all serve the same function. The oestrogen in HT is generally synthesised from an active ingredient called diosgenin, which is a molecule extracted from various plants including wild yam, and has the ability to be converted into either oestrogen or progesterone in a lab. Another source of oestrogen is from the urine of pregnant horses, known as Premarin. Why horses you may ask? – Basically because horses are big and pee a lot, and their oestrogen rich urine is readily available. Progestogen is the synthetic form of progesterone which is most commonly used in HT, mainly because the bio-identical form of progesterone is poorly absorbed in tablet form; however, it can be very effective when used in topical applications. There are many varieties of progestogen, but they all have the same essential function in HT, which is to protect the lining of the uterus.

Hormones Used
Natural oestrogen (estradiol, estrone and estriol) - Derived from plant and animal origin
Synthetic oestrogen (ethinyl estradiol and mestranol) – Synthetic oestrogen produced in lab

Natural oestrogens tend to cause fewer side effects as the body is able to process them more effectively.

Bio-identical progesterone - chemically identical to natural progesterone but created in a lab from plant origin (mainly used in trans- dermal applications).

Synthetic progesterone - (progestins) synthetic compound that mimics most activity of progesterone, but does not have the same chemical structure.

Progestogen - combination of naturally occurring and synthetic progesterone as well synthetic progestins.

The Three Main Types of HT are:

Cyclical HT

This is recommended to women who are experiencing menopausal symptoms but still have their periods. There are two types of cyclical HT:

Monthly - when you take oestrogen every day and progesterone or a progestin at the end of your monthly cycle for 14 days.

Tri Monthly - where you take oestrogen every day and also take progesterone or a progestin for 14 days every 13 weeks.

Monthly HT is normally recommended for women who are having regular periods and the tri monthly HT is recommended for women who have irregular periods.

Oestrogen Only HT

This is usually recommended for post-menopausal women who have had their uterus and ovaries removed (hysterectomy). As you no longer have a uterus, you are no longer at risk of developing endometrial cancer or cancer of the uterine lining.

Continuous Combined HT

Recommended for women who are post-menopausal, and as the name suggests, includes taking oestrogen and progesterone/progestin continuously ever day without a break.

Combined HT is available in various forms including:

- Tablets
- Patches
- Skin Gels
- Implants

Combined HT can also be administered vaginally with creams, rings or suppositories, or for progesterone only via an intrauterine device (IUD).
You would normally take HT for two to three years. Some women find that symptoms return for a short time after stopping HT.

Taking HT for a long time may slightly increase the risks of developing:
- Breast cancer
- Endometrial cancer
- Deep vein thrombosis
- Gall stones
- Strokes and possible heart diseases

The Women's Health Initiative Study has found that after five years of use, combined HT is associated with an overall 26 percent increase in risk of breast cancer. The risk with oestrogen-only HT is not significantly increased.
The Million Women Study has found that for women aged 50 who do not use HT, about 32 in every thousand will develop breast cancer by the time they reach the age of 65 years. If women take an oestrogen-only preparation between ages 50 to 65 for five years, the total number of cases would be between 33 and 34 in every thousand (i.e. an extra one to two cases). If they take it for 10 years, there would be 37 in a thousand (i.e. an extra five cases).

While there are risks associated with HT, most experts agree that if used on a short term basis, for no more than five years, the benefits can outweigh the risks.

Bio-identical Hormones
Many women still have reservations about taking HT and as a consequence of this, interest has grown in bio-identical hormones. Bio-identical hormones sound more appealing when dealing with the menopause because they are derived naturally, and our bodies can metabolise them properly because they are identical to our own hormones. There are two categories of bio-identical hormones: preparations pre-made and distributed by major pharmaceutical companies and those made up in a compounding pharmacy, which are custom-made and specifically designed to match your individual

hormone needs. Both kinds can be created in a number of forms, including pills, creams, patches, and gels as well as vaginal rings.

Bio-identical hormone therapy is often referred to as 'natural', but the word 'natural' can be quite misleading. Companies can advertise their hormone products as being 'natural' because they are from a plant origin, but all hormones, whether from plant origin or not, have to go through a chemical process, effectively making them synthesised. The only true, natural hormones are the ones your own body makes.

Bio-identical hormones - are manufactured in a lab from synthesised plant or animal ingredients. They are chemically identical to the hormones produced by a woman's body.

Non-bio-identical hormones - are also manufactured in a lab using synthesised ingredients, derived from plant or animal sources. But they are not chemically identical to the hormones produced by a woman's body.

Synthetic hormones – are technically any hormones not produced by a woman's body. Even if the hormones are derived from plant sources, they still have to be synthesised in a lab.

When you take a Bio-Identical hormone, your body cannot tell the difference between the hormone molecules it made and the hormones you take; they will have the same elements, chemical bonds, shape, and chemical activity. This applies to bio-identical progesterone, testosterone, and other hormones too.
However, it's important to remember that no drug, supplement or herb is 100 percent safe - there is always a chance that you may experience an adverse reaction.
If bio-identical hormone therapy is something you are interested in, then we recommend that you consult with your doctor or a hormone

specialist before beginning any treatment to safe-guard you from side effects.

Testosterone/Androgen Therapy
You may be prescribed testosterone if an insufficiency is suspected. It will be combined with oestrogen and progesterone or progestin, as taking it on its own may cause adverse effects. This hormone is given to treat hot flushes if oestrogen is not enough. Long term risks are not known, but too large a dose could result in aggression, acne, excessive facial hair, lowering of the voice and muscle and weight gain.

Take the time to decide if HT is for you. No two women are the same, what suits you may not suit another. If you do decide to go ahead with it you may need to play around a little with the doses and combinations until you find one that suits you. Do not hesitate to go back to your doctor if it's not meeting your requirements, and keep going back until it's right.

Adrenal Glands

During the menopause we know our ovarian oestrogen and progesterone levels drop, giving rise to many of the symptoms we are all too familiar with.
However, other body areas are still capable of producing these hormones. One of the most important is the adrenal glands. These two small glands sit at the top of the kidneys and are responsible for producing our sex hormones from cholesterol.
As the ovarian functions diminish and hormone levels drop off during menopause, the pituitary gland sends signals to the adrenals to increase their hormone output and these glands should then replace what was lost from the ovaries.
Unfortunately many women today suffer from under activity of the adrenal glands, caused by stress, nutritional deficiency and lifestyle choices, making it difficult for the body to respond and adapt to this

new need for hormones.

Strong adrenal glands encourage a more balanced menopause, so it is important to keep them in a healthy state. Certain herbs can actually help to stimulate the body's own hormonal production and support the adrenal glands, thus gradually normalising hormonal levels, and gently alleviating menopause symptoms ,without the need for hormone replacement therapy.

Maca root is one of the most popular herbs for helping to balance the adrenal glands. Unlike other HT remedies, Maca does not supply the body with hormones. It is a non-oestrogenic herb and instead it nurtures the adrenal glands, prompting them to create natural hormones. So, whether your body is producing too much or too little of a particular hormone, by using Maca, your system will get back into a balanced state, and symptoms of menopause such as night sweats, hot flushes, vaginal dryness and sleeplessness may be significantly reduced.

You should see your doctor or qualified herbalist for professional advice on adrenal functions and helping to support them.

Alternatively, you will find some remedies available in health shops and in the Phytomone range of supplements, where the Maca root is used to help to support hormonally changing skin and to balance the adrenal glands.

Medical Matters

Bleeding

Most women will experience some changes in bleeding patterns during peri-menopause. It is normal to miss periods, to have lighter or heavier bleeding or for periods to be longer or shorter in duration. It is also normal for these irregular patterns to carry on all the way through peri-menopause, until bleeding stops for good.

What is Abnormal Bleeding?

If you have any of the following symptoms during peri-menopause you should talk to your doctor to confirm it is not associated with any other health problems. He will want to give you a complete examination to exclude any serious causes. This will involve a vaginal examination, cervical smear and blood tests for anaemia and thyroid function. You may also be referred for an ultra sound examination of the pelvic organs.

Very heavy bleeding (using several pads over an hour) particularly when accompanied by clots.
The most serious possible cause is cancer of the uterus, known as endometrial cancer. More likely than not there will be a simple explanation, so don't automatically assume it is a sign of cancer.

Bleeding that lasts for more than five days in a row, or when the interval between periods becomes shorter (less than 21 days).
This may be due to fibroids, polyps, endometrial hyperplasia and VERY rarely endometrial cancer.

Continual spotting or bleeding that begins after you've had intercourse.
This could be due to an infection in the uterus or fallopian tubes or there is a very small chance it could be cancer of the cervix.

Bleeding with severe pain
Probably an infection or fibroid related problem.

Bleeding with a high temperature
Most likely to be an infection.

Gauging Your Blood Flow

Spotting
A drop or two of blood, not even requiring sanitary protection (though you may prefer to use some).

Very Light Bleeding
Requires changing of sanitary protection only one or two times a day.

Light Bleeding
Requires changing of sanitary protection two or three times and day.

Moderate Bleeding

Requires changing a regular-absorbency pad or tampon every three to four hours.

Heavy Bleeding

Requires using a high-absorbency pad or tampon, changing every three to four hours.

Very Heavy Bleeding

Sanitary protection hardly works at all. You need to use the highest-absorbency pad or tampon and change every hour.

What is Menstrual Fluid?

It is a combination of cervical mucus, cells from the uterine lining, vaginal secretions and blood.

Bleeding Terminology

Amenorrhea

When periods have stopped, temporarily or permanently.

Hypomenorrhea

Light periods that are considered to be below average blood loss but appear at regular intervals.

Oligomenorrhea

Periods are light, irregular or infrequent.

Dysmenorrhea

Periods have become painful - medical term for menstrual cramps.

Metorrhagia

Bleeding is occurring between menstrual periods.

Menometrorrhagia

Periods are often heavy and occur more frequently and irregularly than normal.

Menorrhagia

Abnormally heavy and prolonged periods at regular intervals.

Bleeding After Menopause

Any bleeding that occurs once you are post-menopausal should be checked out by a doctor.

This bleeding could be nothing and may just be due to the fact you are still producing small amounts of oestrogen, or you may have an infection that requires antibiotics.

However, in a very small number of cases it could be a warning sign of a gynaecological cancer. So it is important to report it to your doctor who will carry out a pelvic examination and may arrange for you to have an ultrasound or biopsy.

Only occasionally does heavy or irregular bleeding signal cancer of the uterus or cervix. But this is the main warning sign of these cancers. Don't automatically assume it's cancer, but for your own peace of mind it is worth getting it checked out.

Endometrial Cancer

This is the most common of the gynaecological cancers and largely targets post-menopausal women. The exact cause is unknown, though increased levels of oestrogen appear to play a role. This cancer is most commonly diagnosed between the ages 50 to 70. Which may seem slightly incongruous, as this is the time when a woman's oestrogen levels are at their lowest. But if a woman was oestrogen dominant in her earlier years then this may have had some effect.

Because the most frequent symptom of endometrial cancer is post-menopausal bleeding, it is usually caught early and most women survive.

Symptoms

Any vaginal bleeding or spotting in post-menopausal women.
Very heavy bleeding or abnormal bleeding during peri-menopause.
Abdominal pain or discomfort.

Pain during intercourse.
Clear or pinkish watery discharge from the vagina.

Cervical Cancer

Develops in the cervix, the opening between the vagina and the uterus. Most cervical cancer is caused by a virus called human papillomavirus (HPV). Having sexual contact with someone who is infected can transmit HPV. There are many types of the HPV virus and not all types cause cervical cancer.

Symptoms

There are often no noticeable symptoms during the early stages of this disease. But be aware of the following signs and mention them to your doctor if necessary:
Heavy bleeding, spotting, and bleeding between periods or after intercourse.
Pain during intercourse.
Foul smelling or pink tinged discharge.
Painful urination.
Pelvic, leg and back pain.

Fibroids

Are non-cancerous tumours that grow in the muscles of the uterus. Symptoms can include prolonged heavy periods accompanied by cramps, painful intercourse, back pain and bladder and bowel problems.
Fibroids tend to shrink and cause fewer problems after menopause due to lower oestrogen levels preventing their growth, but if they are very troublesome during peri-menopause they can be surgically removed.

Breast Cancer

A woman's risk of developing breast cancer is related to her cumulative exposure to oestrogen as well as her breast sensitivity to the hormone.
For example, if you started menstruating at a young age, say before 12 and your menopause started late, after 55, you will have been exposed to more oestrogen compared to the woman whose periods started later and reached menopause earlier.
Women who have never been pregnant, or become pregnant for the

first time after the age of 30 are also at increased risk, as they were exposed to more oestrogen when they were young.

In addition, breast tissue has the ability to concentrate, produce and metabolise oestrogen, and there is often 10 to 40 times more oestrogen in the breasts than the level circulating in the blood. Oestrogen interacts with breast tissue through oestrogen receptors, which are proteins in the cells that act like docking stations for the oestrogen circulating in your body. When oestrogen docks at a receptor, it can encourage the cell to proliferate. Most of the time cell division produces healthier breast tissue. But cells that contain cancer causing mutations can proliferate and grow to become tumours. Though not all tumours are sensitive to oestrogen, oestrogen may cause changes in cells that can eventually lead to cancer.

Most women who get breast cancer are over 65, which doesn't seem to make a lot of sense since by this time oestrogen levels have plummeted. But experts believe that ageing cells are more likely to have DNA damage due to a lifetime of exposure to toxins, disease, weight gain and lifestyle choices and as a result, make more cell division errors and create more abnormal versions of themselves. Breast cancer is generally slow growing and often takes a while to show itself. So, although oestrogen levels are now low, the damage has already been done and your immune system, which has also weakened over time, is less able to fight off the cancer.

Symptoms
A lump or area of thickening in the breast.
Change in size or shape.
Dimpling or puckering of the skin.
Nipple becomes turned in.
Swelling or lump in the armpit.
Any discharge (clear or bloody) from the nipple.

Mammograms
You want to do everything you can as early as possible to find any cancer cells in your body. So it is important to have regular screening, especially after you reach the age of 50. Although mammograms cannot detect all types of cancer, they are still an effective way to detect early cancer. During a mammogram each breast is placed on the x-ray machine and then compressed slightly

with a plastic plate. The x-ray will show if there are any areas of abnormality which need addressing.

Premature Menopause

Premature or early menopause usually occurs before the age of 40. This may be brought on by medical treatments such as chemotherapy or surgery, or it may have no obvious cause.

Being diagnosed with early menopause can be devastating, in particular the loss of fertility if you haven't had any or all the children you want yet.

Women who enter menopause early are at a greater risk for health problems such as osteoporosis or heart disease when they are older, and hormone therapy may be advised to help counteract these risks. The symptoms are generally the same, hot flushes, night sweats, fatigue, dry vagina and so on, except it is all happening a decade or so before it should be. Some women feel emotionally traumatised at being diagnosed with premature menopause and feel their body has let them down in some way, or they blame themselves for bringing it on by some past unhealthy behaviour. In fact the cause of premature menopause is still not clear. Genetics or an autoimmune disease could be the cause, but most women never learn why their ovaries stopped functioning. However, some disease and conditions are associated with premature menopause and these are:

- Thyroid disease
- Hypoparathyroidism
- Rheumatoid Arthritis
- Diabetes
- Vitiligo
- Lupus
- Fragile X Syndrome
- Adrenal Insufficiency

Much more information can be found at www.daisynetwork.org

Therapeutic Approach and Complementary Therapy

Herbal Treatments

Black Cohosh
This is one of the most popular herbal treatments for menopause. Black cohosh is anti-inflammatory and has oestrogen like properties, making it an effective herbal treatment for hot flushes, night sweats, vaginal dryness and muscle pain.

Studies of its effectiveness have mixed results, and there is no scientific evidence to back up any claims. But if it is helping your symptoms you don't really need any proof in the form of scientific evidence; if it's working for you, that's all that matters. However, do be aware that links have been made between black cohosh and the risk of liver disorder. From now on will carry a safety warning to this effect.

Black cohosh also contains salicylates which are naturally occurring chemicals in plants that act as a preservative to prevent rotting and defend against harmful bacteria. Certain drugs or compounds are derived from salicylic acid - such as aspirin - so if you are already taking aspirin or other blood thinners you should not use black cohosh.

Dong Quai
Is a native perennial plant from south west China and is currently used in Chinese medicine for thinning the blood. Menopausal women use it for hot flushes and cramps.

Due to its blood thinning properties women with fibroids, haemophilia or other blood clotting disorders should not use this herbal treatment.

Evening Primrose Oil
Is a very rich source of gamma linolenic acid (omega 6 fatty acid) and can help some women with symptoms of hot flushes and mood swings; it also appear to be useful for mastalgia (breast pain/tenderness).

Ginkgo Biloba
Is thought to have a beneficial effect on cognitive impairment such as confusion, forgetfulness, brain fog and dementia and also promotes a sense of well-being. It appears to be relatively safe with only mild side effects reported such as headaches and nausea.

Ginseng
Can improve energy levels, relieve stress and mood symptoms. It can stimulate low sex drive and boost immunity. Side effects can include headaches, dizziness, hypertension and inhibit platelet aggregation (blood clotting). Do not combine with aspirin or anti-coagulants.

St. Johns Wort
Has an anti-depressant effect and reduces anxiety by inhibiting the neurotransmitters in the brain. It is also a popular treatment for sleep disorders and helps ease feelings of low spirits and loss of self-esteem. Do not use if you are taking heart medication or other anti-depressants (especially SSRI's) or the birth control pill.

Chasteberry
Thought to have a hormone regulating effect and may be helpful during peri-menopause. Women have reported improvements in moods and headaches but there is little scientific evidence to support this.

Sage
Can give relief from hot flushes. Drink fresh sage leaves made into a tea or use a concentrated formula, adding a few drops to a glass of water.

Liquorice
Helps to balance oestrogen and progesterone. Liquorice root tea may help with mood swings, hot flushes, irregular periods, vaginal dryness and sore breasts. It may also help to maintain energy levels.
To make liquorice tea:
1 teaspoon liquorice root powder
8oz. boiling water
Steep for 4-7 minutes

Red Clover
Contains oestrogen like compounds and can help with hot flushes, vaginal dryness, mood swings and osteoporosis, and has the ability to cleanse and thin the blood, though scientific evidence is lacking. It has mild anti-coagulant properties so avoid if you are taking aspirin or pharmaceutical anti-coagulants. Do not take if you are oestrogen dominant.

Gotu Kola
Used to help counteract loss of memory and mental function. Not to be used in pregnancy or by people who suffer from epilepsy.

Valerian
Appears to have a sedative effect and may help with sleep disorders. There are no known side effects.

Nettle Leaves
Either drink as an infusion or eat as a green vegetable. Like seaweed, they are extremely nourishing to the entire endocrine system. Among other things they are a good source of calcium, magnesium, chlorophyll, chromium, plus many other minerals and vitamins. Two cups a day is recommended.

Alfalfa
Take as a tablet, tea or eat in salads. Helps to promote oestrogen production if your levels are low.

Oats
Whether eaten or infused they will nourish and help balance your hormonal system. An infusion of oat straw will also have the same benefits.

Therapies

Acupuncture and Acupressure
Acupuncture uses needles put into the skin at specific points in the body.

Acupressure uses pressure on these same points.

These points correspond to our energy (chi) channels, also known as 'meridians', which are believed to link to internal organs and unblock energy and balance the flow, helping to correct illnesses and psychological problems.

Studies show that acupuncture can be beneficial in treating hot flushes, night sweats, joint pain, lower back pain and arthritis.

Hypnotherapy

Aims to improve health through inducing a trance-like state. It has been useful to treat symptoms of stress and anxiety, but to date there are no reports on the benefits of hypnotherapy being used for other menopausal symptoms.

Aromatherapy

Is the use of concentrated plant oils to treat illnesses and ailments. The oils can be applied through massage, inhalation or in the bath. More details on aromatherapy can be found in the Body and Soul Chapter of this book.

Reflexology

Uses the energy channels and meridians similar to those in acupuncture and acupressure, but these are contained within the feet. It is a gentle technique which aims to restore and maintain the body's natural equilibrium, by stimulating the reflex points on the feet which correspond to the organs in the body. Reflexology can be effective for back pain, migraine, sleep disorders, hormone imbalance and stress related conditions.

Homeopathy and TCM (Traditional Chinese Medicine)

Aims to cure like with like and stimulate the body into healing itself. Homeopathic remedies have been demonstrated to reduce hot flushes and to improve quality of life. Traditional homeopathic practitioners select and administer a remedy based on a woman's symptoms and physical, mental and emotional state. This then strengthens the body's vital defences and restores a healthy balance and sense of well-being. Most of the major homeopathic remedies may be used to treat symptoms of menopause.

Some scientists believe that the dilution of homeopathic preparations is so great that no active ingredients remain in the remedies prescribed, and insist the positive effects are caused by the placebo effect. However, homeopathic treatments have been used successfully for the past two hundred years, so if it works for you then it is good enough.

Massage
A relaxing therapy that will improve the lymphatic system and blood circulation, bringing the body back into harmony and helping to soothe your mind and nourish your soul.

Yoga
Is considered to be a moving form of meditation and is a wonderful activity to add to your routine. It helps relieve stress, prevent mood swings, increase strength and flexibility, and ward off osteoporosis.

Meditation and Breathing Techniques
Will help you focus and calm your mind. These techniques will give you an overall sense of well-being which in turn helps you manage your menopausal symptoms in a much more positive way.
More techniques can be found in the Body and Soul Chapter.

Phytomone Spa Therapy Products
A range of body care products specifically designed for hormonally changing skin.
The products have been developed with the perfect balance of the most effective herbs for menopausal symptoms.

- Bath Crystals
- Body Oil/Serum
- Shower Gel
- Exfoliating Soap Bar
- Face Cream
- Face Cleansing Oil
- Body Cream
- Cooling Body Powder
- Cooling Spray
- Dry Shower Powder

Chapter Two

EXERCISE

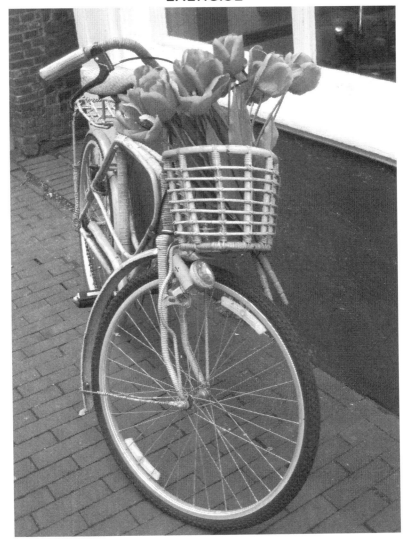

Why Exercise and What Your Changing Body Requires

The benefits of regular exercise during menopause are huge.Some research suggests that women who are physically active may have fewer menopausal symptoms.

But the truth of the matter is most of us don't have the time or the desire to include exercise into our daily routine.
So, before we even begin exercising we have to change our mental attitude. The first thing you need to do is make time in your day and book yourself in for a regular appointment to exercise, whether it's at the gym, club, pool or at home, and just make sure you don't cancel it any more than you would your doctor's or dentist appointment - this is just as important and not really an option.
You don't have to train to run the next marathon or spend hours in the gym; this is about finding a routine that's right for you and tailoring it to suit your needs for this stage of your life. Research continues to show that 20 to 30 minutes of exercise a day not only helps you live longer, but stay healthier too.Better still, it doesn't have to be done all at once - 10 minutes at a time is fine as long as you are doing the activity at a moderate or vigorous level.
You could try going for a brisk 10 minute walk three times a day for example. Of course this may not suit you and you may prefer to do your work out all in one go, but this just gives you the option to adapt a convenient routine to suit your lifestyle.
The most important thing, and probably the hardest, is being committed. We all start out with a very positive attitude, but it's not long before the focus diminishes and we start to find reasons and excuses why we can't do our workout today. This is the hard part because you have to be mentally strong and strict with yourself.
Unless it's a major emergency there is no reason why you shouldn't do your exercises, so stop trying to justify your excuse.
Once you have worked through that 'wobbly stage' of giving up and you're in the habit of doing your exercises, along with all of your other daily commitments and chores, you will have no desire to go back to your old ways.You will feel so much better in both physical

strength and mental well-being, and probably feel quite proud of yourself too.

During menopause and post menopause we are more at risk of developing

- Osteoporosis
- Heart Disease
- High Blood Pressure
- Decreased Metabolism
- Weight Gain
- Loss of Muscle Mass
- Loss of Balance

We need to be mentally and physically strong enough to deal with all the challenges menopause throws at us, such as hot flushes and night sweats, muscle aches and pains, mood swings, memory loss, lack of energy and lack of sleep.
We need to get those endorphins flowing and the 'feel good' factor in place and put the 'fizz' back into our life. Middle age does not mean you're a 'has been'; it's the next stage of your life,when you have the luxury to put yourself first, think about you and enjoy some quality time.
But in order to do all of this and take full advantage of this time, you need to be as fit as a fiddle. Embracing a regular exercise routine now, will be your insurance policy to a better quality of life and a healthier future.

"Old age is no place for sissies" – Bettie Davis

Benefits of Exercise

- Strengthens heart muscles
- Builds muscle mass
- Increases bone density
- Lowers blood pressure
- Improves strength and endurance
- Strengthens bones and ligaments
- Improves metabolism
- Improves digestion

- Burns calories/weight loss
- Lowers cholesterol levels
- Improves posture
- Improves self-esteem
- Makes you feel happy
- Gives a healthy glow
- Improves balance
- Quicker recovery from accidents

With so many benefits to help counteract menopausal symptoms, now is the time to embark on your new exercise regime and improve the quality of your new life.

So, it's 'game-on' ladies! Let's work with what we've got and make the most of everything we have!

What Your Changing Body Requires

We Need To:
Increase cardiovascular and respiratory capacity
Increase muscle mass and strength
Increase flexibility and improve balance

Cardio -Vascular (Aerobic)

These exercises include any activity that gets you breathing harder and your heart beating faster. The point is to make your heart stronger and increase the amount of blood it is able to pump with each stroke, and to decrease your pulse rate while at rest.

Aerobic (meaning 'with oxygen') exercises fall into this category. They are good for lowering blood pressure because of their continual use of the circulatory system, which helps reduce cholesterol levels and also build resistance to stress, all significant in reducing the risk of heart attacks and strokes.

Aerobic exercises will help speed up your metabolism and burn calories, as well as increasing your lung capacity, by expanding to allow in more oxygen as you exercise and remove waste carbon more efficiently, so you will not get out of breath so quickly.

Cardio workouts involve using the body's largest muscle groups in a repetitive way over a period of time. In fact you may be surprised at how much aerobic exercise is already incorporated into your everyday routine. By increasing the intensity of how you approach them, you can increase the health benefits substantially. Activities that would otherwise be merely 'calorie burning' can become officially aerobic. In other words, they would be strenuous enough to raise the heart rate and oxygen consumption to levels capable of improving fitness. So, take a look at your daily routine and put a little more 'oomph' into your day. Many types of activities count, from pushing the lawn mower, vacuuming, cleaning windows, to washing the car. As long as you are doing them at a moderate or vigorous intensity for at least 10 minutes at a time you will gain some benefit.

I'm afraid light daily activities such as cooking or doing the laundry don't count because your body isn't working hard enough to get your heart rate up.

Other aerobic/cardio-vascular exercises include:

- General aerobics
- Brisk walking or jogging
- Water aerobics
- Swimming laps
- Playing tennis
- Stair climbing

- Treadmill
- Cross Trainer
- Cycling
- Ice-Skating

Or if you're feeling adventurous how about water-skiing, surfing, rollerblading or even trampolining. Where ever you live and whatever your lifestyle there will be a variety of aerobic exercises available. Just remember whatever activity you choose, it should raise your heart rate and break a sweat.

Talk Test

An easy way of assessing whether you have reached aerobic level is to try and sing your favourite song. You will probably be able to talk the words, but have difficulty singing them.

Benefits Of Cardio-Vascular/Aerobic Exercise

- Improves heart function
- Reduces risk of heart disease
- Reduces risk of osteoporosis
- Improves muscle tone
- Relieves stress
- Helps with weight management
- Increases lung capacity
- Improves mood
- Helps you sleep better
- Improves stamina

Muscle Strengthening and Endurance

Of course there is more to exercise than just a healthy heart - we also need some muscle power to go with it.

As we age and go through menopause we lose muscle mass, so it is important to add strength building exercises to our routine to restore muscle tissue and tighten up those flabby arms, jelly bellies and wobbly bottoms and thighs.

Stronger muscles will have a positive effect on your normal daily activities, giving you both strength and endurance to carry on just that little bit longer, whether it's gardening, carrying heavy bags back from the supermarket, completing your exercise routine or just being able to undo the lid on that jar of marmalade.

Muscle is also important for weight control, because muscle is the best calorie burning tissue we have. It is more effective than fat even when at rest, so the more muscle we have the better at burning calories we are going to be, even if we are just watching the TV.

It is commonly misunderstood that fat can be turned into muscle. Fat and muscle are two distinctly different tissues and one cannot be turned into the other. Muscle will always be muscle and fat will always be fat. Body fat is a storage place where our body puts extra energy when we consume more calories per day than we burn off. When we 'burn fat' we are actually shrinking the size of our fat cells by using the energy that has been stored there, so you are not actually losing fat, your fat cells are just getting smaller (fat cells are capable of expanding up to a thousand times their original size). Muscle, on the other hand, is an active tissue that moves and burns calories around the clock, and by stimulating muscle through exercise we are building and strengthening their connective fibre. This in turn requires energy that we get from our stored energy supply, like fat cells, so by exercising you will be burning the fat and building the muscle.

Fast Twitch and Slow Twitch Fibres

Our muscle tissue is composed of two types of fibres: fast twitch and slow twitch.

When we exercise aerobically we are using our slow twitch fibres. These fibres gain in endurance from continuous rhythmic aerobic exercise, but they do not increase in strength, so you could run a marathon but not necessarily lift heavy weights no matter how much you trained.

On the other hand, our fast twitch fibres get called into action when we exercise in a strength building way. Muscle builders focus on their fast twitch fibres and amazing growth can be the result, but though they have the strength it will only be in short bursts and would not have the endurance of a marathon runner.

One thing to remember here is, as we age studies show we lose muscle mass and strength almost entirely due to atrophy of our fast twitch muscle fibres and not our slow twitch. This is because our slow twitch fibres get called upon by even the most minimum exertions, and by contrast our fast twitchers do very little as we age, and can eventually disappear if we neglect them.

Strength building exercises will add good muscular firmness and shape. They should be done at least three or four times a week and work all the major muscle groups of your body (legs, hips, back, chest, abdomen, shoulders and arms).

We need to exercise the larger muscle groups first so we don't exhaust the smaller muscle groups, that are also needed to exercise the larger muscles.

Because strength exercises can be used to target different muscle groups, you might like to choose to concentrate say, on your arms one day and work on your legs the next. However, after a good workout session you should rest the muscles exercised for 24 hours, as they need this time to respond to the stimulus and build up additional mass.

Major Muscle Groups

All muscles work in pairs to provide movement and stability. The pairs are located opposite one another. When one muscle contracts the other relaxes; for example, when your bicep muscles in your upper arm contract, they pull your lower arm in towards your shoulder and your tricep muscles on the underside of your upper arm contracts and straightens your arm out again.

Muscle Strengthening Exercises

- Weight Training
- Resistance Training
- Calisthenics (using your own body weight for resistance)
- Pilates
- Tai Chi
- Yoga

Resistance Aids

Use dumbbells for added weight.
Ankle and wrist weights will increase the amount of resistance, use when doing strength-training exercises.
Elastic training bands increase resistance when used in some straight forward exercises at home.
Gym machines used for workouts.
Barbells .

Benefits

- Builds muscles
- Improves co-ordination
- Burns calories
- Improves flexibility
- Raises metabolism
- Wards off osteoporosis and arthritis
- Increases strength and endurance
- Improves self esteem

Stretching and Balance

As we age our tendons and ligaments begin to shorten and tighten, it is important to keep our muscle joints flexible and mobile so we can move through a full range of motions and avoid discomforts such as muscle tension and painful joints.

Stretching can stimulate the production of lubricants between the connective tissue fibres, helping to alleviate some of the side effects of both ageing and the menopausal transition.

Stretching is one way to keep the body flexible, but it is important to warm up before you start, to reduce the risk of injury; warm muscles are more pliable than cold ones.

Stretching exercises will also improve balance and co-ordination, something we definitely need to pay more attention to as we age.

You can test your balance by seeing how long you can stand on one leg. Lift one leg just slightly off the ground and hold your balance for as long as possible. You may need to hold on to a chair or use the wall to keep steady initially. When you feel more confident, try balancing by yourself, or by placing only your fingertips on the surface, and gradually work towards not holding on at all. Finally when you have mastered this techniqu,e try it with your eyes closed. Be sure to have something or someone close by to hold on to though - should you need to.

Exercises
- General stretching
- Yoga
- Pilates
- Tai Chi

Benefits

- Increases co-ordination and balance
- Keeps muscles supple and flexible
- Can help reduce stress
- Develops body awareness
- Reduces pain in joints and muscles
- Reduces risk of injuries
- Feels relaxing

So remember you need to include all three types of exercise in your routine:

Cardio-Vascular-Aerobic
Muscle Strengthening
Stretching and Balance

Aim to exercise every day for at least 20 to 30 minutes
Do muscle-strengthening exercises every other day to allow muscles to build up additional mass.
Mix and match you exercises - variety will keep your muscles guessing about what is coming next and will also stop you from becoming bored with your work-out routine. Make sure you choose something you enjoy or be adventurous and try something new.

Aerobic Exercise

- Running
- Brisk Walking
- Swimming Laps
- Cycling
- Dancing
- Housework
- Tennis
- Skating
- Golf
- Gardening

Muscle Strengthening Exercise

- Weight training
- Resistance training
- Calisthenics
- Pilates
- Tai Chi
- Yoga

Stretching Exercise

- General stretching
- Balance exercise
- Tai Chi
- Yoga

How To Find Your Maximum Heart Rate

For an adult, a normal resting heart rate ranges from 60 to 100 beats a minute. For a well-trained athlete, a normal resting heart rate may be closer to 40 beats a minute. For healthy adults, a lower heart rate at rest generally implies more efficient heart function and better cardiovascular fitness.

You can assess your fitness level by finding out what your maximum heart rate is (MHR).
Work this out by subtracting your age from 220
For example if you are 56 it would be:
$220 - 56 = 164$
This is the upper limit of what your Heart Rate can handle during a workout.

Target Heart Rate

This will show you if you are working hard and putting enough energy into your routine to reap the benefits.
Calculate it at 60% - 80% of your maximum heart rate
Beginners calculate the formula at 60%
When the routine becomes easier move up to 70%
As you get stronger move up to 80%

So for example if your MHR is 164 and you are just beginning an exercise routine the sum would be $164 \times .60 = 98.4$

This is your target heart rate of beats per minute and what you should be aiming for. If you are not achieving this then you need to push yourself a little harder to get the maximum results and to see and feel the benefits.

THR =Target Heart Rate

Beginners:
Maximum Heart Rate x .60 = THR
Intermediate:
Maximum Heart Rate x .70 = THR
Advanced:
Maximum Heart Rate x .80 = THR

Example of Weekly Workout Routine

Mon - Full Body Workout 45-60 mins.
Tues - Aerobics and Stretching 20-30 mins.
Wed - Muscle Strengthening and Stretching 20-30 mins.
Thu - Aerobics and Stretching 20-30 mins.
Fri - Muscle Strengthening and Stretching 20-30 mins.
Sat - Aerobics and Stretching 20-30 mins.
Sun - Muscle Strengthening and Stretching 20-30 mins.

Remember you can mix and match and choose different exercises from the different groups. Choose one day a week where you have a full-body work-out. Monday is good as it sets you up for the week ahead, and then alternate your muscle strengthening exercises with your aerobic exercise. You can of course do aerobic exercises every day if you wish, but make sure you only do your muscle-strengthening exercises every other day; this gives them time to respond to the stimulus and then you can increase the weights when you no longer find them difficult.

Menopause Full Body Workout Programme (coming soon)

We have put together this set of exercises specifically for the transition through menopause and into post menopause.
It is a full body workout and includes some effective exercises for strength, endurance, flexibility and balance.
The exercises are rhythmic and sustained so they provide cardiovascular conditioning, and you will be using your own body weight for the muscle strengthening exercises.

We will begin with the warm-up to raise the pulse rate and prepare the muscles for the main workout.
The main workout will consist of aerobic, muscle strengthening, flexibility and balance exercises.
Finally we will 'cool down' with a set of low impact exercises which gradually return the body to its resting state. This will help to get rid of any metabolic waste products that may have accumulated during the exercise session.
During exercise blood is being pumped around the body by the heart and then returned back to the heart by the venous system and muscular contractions. If you stop exercising suddenly, the heart continues to beat fast, sending blood around the body, but because the exercise has stopped, the blood is no longer assisted in its return to the heart. This is known as 'blood pooling' by athletes and may be one reason why you may feel faint after exercising.
It's very important to always do a cool down after exercising and to allow the heart to gradually return to its resting level.

Preparing for Your Workout

Try to set a regular time, write it on your calendar, just like you would any other appointment, and don't cancel it! By having a specific time put aside to exercise you are more likely to do it rather than just trying to fit it in somewhere in your day. Remember exercise is important for your pain-free future.

Make sure you won't be disturbed during your exercise and switch your phone off.

If you are exercising at home make sure you have a place where there is enough room to swing your arms and kick your legs.

You will need an exercise pad or towel to give you a little padding for the floor work.

Wear comfortable clothing.

A big mirror is great to exercise in front of - but not essential.

Music may help you along the way. Experiment with what you like and work with it.

If you are not used to exercising don't push yourself too hard to begin with or you may get hurt. Once you can do all the reps without strain, add some weight and increase the reps.

Remember to breathe correctly; this will increase your oxygen intake and improve circulation, helping to get rid of toxins.

Supplementary Exercises
(Anytime Exercises)

Buttock Crunch
Stand tall, tummy tucked in, shoulders back. Now simply contract the muscles in your buttocks, hold for 20 seconds, breathe normally, release and repeat throughout the day.

Pelvic Floor Exercises
Strengthening the muscles in the pelvic floor is one way to gain control of the bladder. As we age our pelvic floor muscles weaken, which can cause urine leakage from the bladder. Try these exercises to help strengthen the pelvic floor.

To find the muscles that control the flow of urine, stop and start your urine next time you go to the bathroom, these are the muscles that you need to work on.

Try tightening them for about five seconds, making sure you use these muscles only. Don't tighten your tummy muscles or your buttocks. Do this exercise throughout the day - no one will know, and try to build up to 20 at a time. It may take a while so be patient with yourself. Just like any other muscle it takes time to build up strength and endurance.

Thigh Squeeze

Sit on a chair, straight backed, both feet flat on the floor and knees bent at a 90 degree angle. Put a pillow between your thighs and squeeze it tightly. Exhale deeply with each squeeze. Hold each squeeze for 30 seconds, building up to one minute. Release and repeat five times.

Thigh Squeeze Two

Sitting on a chair put palms of hands on outside of knees. Push knees outwards as if trying to push your hands away, at the same time push inwards with your hands as if you're trying to push your knees together. Hold for one minute and repeat three times. This works the front and outer thighs.

Ankle Flex

Still in the chair, extend right leg out and rotate ankle clockwise 10 times and then anti-clockwise 10 times. Lower leg and repeat with left leg.

Buttock and Thigh Lift

Put your arms out in front of you and raise yourself up from the chair, now lower yourself back down. Repeat 10 times, ending in the standing position.

Wall Squat

Find a free wall and lean back against it. Feet should be shoulder-width apart and a few inches away from the wall. Now slide down the wall until your thighs are parallel with the floor, like you're sitting on an invisible chair. Hold this position for as long as you can then come up into standing position.

Always take the stairs rather than the elevator.

Make a point of walking briskly every day.

High Intensity Interval Training (HIIT)

Losing weight during menopause can sometimes prove difficult. No matter how much you exercise or follow a healthy eating plan, you just can't seem to shed those extra pounds.

You know that your metabolism has slowed down and the lack of oestrogen in your body is making a lot of things harder, and don't forget your fat cells produce a small amount of oestrogen which your body is not too keen to give up.
If you have reached a plateau and feel like you are on a long road to no-where, don't give up just yet because some High Intensity Interval Training might just wake your body up and get things moving.

How It Works
HIIT is a specialised form of interval training that involves short intervals of maximum intensity exercise separated by longer intervals of low to moderate intensity exercise. Because it involves briefly pushing yourself beyond the upper end of your aerobic exercise zone, it offers you several advantages that traditional steady-state exercise (where you keep your heart rate within your aerobic zone) can't provide:

• HIIT trains and conditions both your *anaerobic* and *aerobic* energy systems. You train your anaerobic system with brief, all-out efforts, like when you have to push to make it up a hill, or sprint to catch the bus.

• Increases the amount of calories you burn during your exercise session and afterwards, because it increases the length of time it takes your body to recover from each exercise session.
• Causes metabolic adaptations that enable you to use more fat as fuel under a variety of conditions. This will improve your fat-burning potential.
• Appears to limit muscle loss that can occur with weight loss, in comparison to traditional steady-state cardio exercise of longer duration.
• To get the benefits of HIIT, you need to push yourself past the upper end of your aerobic zone and allow your body to replenish your anaerobic energy system during the recovery intervals.

The key element of HIIT that makes it different from other forms of interval training is that the high intensity intervals involve *maximum* effort, not simply a higher heart rate. There are many different approaches to HIIT, each involving different numbers of high and low intensity intervals, different levels of intensity during the low intensity intervals, different lengths of time for each interval, and different numbers of training sessions per week.

General HIIT Guidelines

• HIIT is designed for people whose primary concerns are boosting overall cardiovascular fitness, endurance, and fat loss, without losing the muscle mass they already have.
• Before starting any HIIT program, you should be able to exercise for at least 20 to 30 minutes at 70 to 85 percent of your estimated maximum heart rate, without exhausting yourself or having problems.
• Because HIIT is physically demanding, it's important to gradually build up your training program so that you don't overdo it. The sample training schedule below will safely introduce you to HIIT over a period of eight weeks.
• Always warm up and cool down for at least five minutes before and after each HIIT session.
• Work as hard as you can during the high intensity intervals, until you feel the burning sensation in your muscles indicating that you have entered your anaerobic zone. Full recovery takes about four minutes for everyone, but you can shorten the recovery intervals if

your high intensity intervals are also shorter and don't completely exhaust your anaerobic energy system.

• If you experience any chest pain or breathing difficulties during your HIIT workout, **cool down** immediately. Don't just stop or else blood can pool in your extremities and light-headedness or faintness can occur.

• If your heart rate does not drop back down to about 70 percent of your maximum during recovery intervals, you may need to shorten your work intervals and/or lengthen your recovery intervals.

• HIIT (including the sample program below) is not for beginner exercisers or people with cardiovascular problems or risk factors. If you have cardiovascular problems or risk factors you should NOT attempt HIIT unless your doctor has specifically cleared you for this kind of exercise.

A Sample Progressive HIIT Program

Week	Warm Up	Work Interval (Max Intensity)	Recovery Interval (60-70% MHR)	Repeat	Cool Down	Total Workout Time
1	5 min.	1 min.	4 min.	2 times	5 min.	20 min.
2	5 min.	1 min.	4 min.	3 times	5 min.	25 min.
3	5 min.	1 min.	4 min.	4 times	5 min.	30 min.
4	5 min.	1.5 min.	4 min.	2 times	5 min.	21 min.
5	5 min.	1.5 min.	4 min.	3 times	5 min.	26.5 min.
6	5 min.	1.5 min.	4 min.	4 times	5 min.	32 min.
7	5 min.	2 min.	5 min.	3 times	5 min.	31 min.
8	5 min.	2 min.	5min.	4 times	5 min.	38 min.

Fig.3

Please adhere to the general HIIT guidelines above for this program. To maximise fat loss, maintain an intensity level of 60-70 percent of your maximum heart rate during warm up, cool down and recovery intervals.

After completing this eight-week program, you can continue working to increase the number of work intervals per session, the duration of work intervals, or both.

You can adjust this training plan to accommodate your particular needs and goals. If you find that this schedule is either too difficult or too easy for your current fitness level, you can make adjustments to the duration and/or number of high intensity intervals as necessary. For example, if you want to train yourself for very short, frequent bursts of maximum intensity activity, your program could involve sprinting for 20 seconds and jogging/walking for 60 seconds, and repeating that 15-20 times per session.

You don't need to swap all of your aerobic exercise for HIIT to gain the benefits. A good balance, for example, might be two sessions of HIIT per week, along with 1-2 sessions of steady-state aerobic exercise. As usual, moderation is the key to long-term success, so challenge yourself—but don't drive yourself into the ground.

HIIT can be applied to all types of cardio equipment and exercise - cross trainers, bikes, and swimming.

Treadmills can be used but you may find they are slow to change speeds, though you can place your feet on either side of the belt while resting if you feel confident enough jumping on and off the machine.

Please remember you will need to have done some regular exercise before you start this program, even at the beginner level.

Even the 'unfit beginner' should be doing some regular form of exercise before starting this training.

Get a physical exam before trying this workout if you have two or more of the following risk factors: a family history of heart disease, you're a smoker, you're sedentary, you're overweight, or you have high cholesterol or high blood pressure.

Hand and Wrist Exercises

Try these exercises to improve flexibility and help aching joints.

Start with the right hand and gently pull back extended fingers one by one.

Now hold your extended fingers together with your left hand and gently pull them all back at the same time. This helps to stretch your palm - Repeat four times.

Stretch your thumb over towards your small finger and then back in the opposite direction.

Now make a tight fist, hold for five seconds and then slowly open it, stretching your fingers and thumb out as far as you can. Repeat on the left hand.

Bring your palms together and elbows out, hold for 30 seconds. Try pushing elbows up towards the ceiling while keeping palms together. Close your eyes and focus on deep breathing.

Open your eyes and stretch your arms forward, fingers pointing straight ahead. Now extend your wrists upwards keeping your arms and fingers straight, hold for five seconds then point your fingers down to the ground without moving your arms and hold for five seconds. Feel the energy pumping forward and out through your wrists.

Finally, keeping your arms still, rotate your wrists in as wide a circle as possible, clockwise eight times and then anti-clockwise eight times.

Relax your arms by your side and loosely shake them.

*If you are suffering from any joint problems such as arthritis, consult your doctor before trying any of the above exercises.

Face Exercises

Facial exercises are a great way of toning the muscles in the face and neck to give a natural lift and a smoother, brighter appearance.
The best results are achieved with regular exercise on a daily basis, so try and get into a routine of doing them at least twice a day.

Double Chin and Jowls
Lift chin towards ceiling and then lower. Repeat 10 times with small slow movements.
Head back, face towards ceiling, and try to kiss the ceiling - hold for five seconds. Repeat five times.
Neck back, open and close mouth while smiling.
Neck back turn to left, push out lower jaw. Repeat five times, change sides and repeat.
Lift chin towards ceiling, push bottom lip up over top lip as far as you can, hold for 10. Repeat five sets.
Head back, teeth together, push tongue up to roof of mouth, hold for 10. Repeat five times.

Cheeks
Place middle two fingers on cheeks and lightly push down, while at the same time trying to raise your cheeks by smiling as hard as you can. Keep your head back while doing this exercise - make sure you

don't apply too much pressure with your fingers, hold for five and repeat five times.

Purse lips, move to the right and then to the left. Repeat 10 times

Put finger in mouth and suck as hard as you can, hold for five and slowly pull out. Repeat five times.

Head back, jaw forward, put upper lip behind lower teeth, smile towards top of ears, hold for five seconds while gently stroking along the jawline. Release and repeat five times.

Eyes

With head back, try to close your eyes by bringing the bottom rim up towards the top eyelid.

Close eyes and relax, look up as far as possible and then down, keeping eyes closed. Repeat five times.

Forehead

Place fingertips under eyebrows and gently lift while at the same time pushing down with your forehead muscles. Repeat five times.

Sit straight, eyes closed, raise eyebrows while at the same time stretching your eyelids down as far as possible by keeping eyes closed.

Healthy Glow Tips

Open your mouth as wide as it will go; feel the stretch in your cheeks, chin and lips, hold and release, repeat five times. This exercise relaxes your facial muscles, increases circulation and relieves tension and stress.

Take a deep breath and exhale forcefully, opening your mouth wide and sticking out your tongue as far as it will go, keep your eyes open and look up. This will relieve tension in the face and throat, improve circulation and stimulate the eyes. Pinch your cheeks by taking flesh into your hands and squeeze **lightly**, this will improve blood circulation.

Brain Fitness

Menopausal women often complain of feeling a little 'spacey' and forgetful and have difficulty concentrating .

Don't worry, you are not alone and you are not going mad. Short-term memory loss is one of the symptoms of menopause, but to date there is no definitive answer as to why.

Some believe it may be due to a drop in oestrogen levels; oestrogen stimulates neurotransmitters, which allow parts of the brain to communicate with one another. Oestrogen also helps dilate blood vessels in the brain, increasing the flow of blood cells that help the brain to function, and a lack of oestrogen could have some effect on this, causing us to be more forgetful.

Natural ageing also causes increased forgetfulness, but it can be exacerbated during menopause by lack of sleep and exhaustion brought on by night sweats, stress, worry and anxiety.

But, take heart ladies, there are many things we can do to improve and maintain brain function. The more our brains are challenged and stimulated, the more receptive they become. Don't worry, you don't have to spend hours working out complicated brain teasers, simple everyday activities are all we need to stay mentally alert.

Recently we have seen a rise in the popularity of the electronic brain games on the market, which are good for stimulation and exercising the grey matter. Don't make the mistake of believing these games can make you more intelligent. To date there is no scientific proof of this, but they do certainly keep you mentally alert and they are fun.

On the other hand, you can also benefit from simply picking up a book, reading newspapers and doing the kind of pencil and paper puzzles that have been available for decades.

We haven't yet learned how to stop the ageing process, but keeping your brain active may help you stay mentally fit while others around you start to fade.

Here are a few ways to improve and re-invigorate your brain with some on-going maintenance.

Ask Why

Our brains are wired to be curious, but as we mature many of us stifle or deny our natural curiosity.

Let yourself be curious, wonder why things are happening, ask questions. The best way to exercise your curiosity is by asking 'why'? Make it a new habit to ask 'why' at least eight times a day. Your brain will be happier and you will be amazed at how many opportunities and solutions will show up.

Memory

Your brain is a memory machine, so improve it and give it chance to work. Try memorising a new poem, or play simple memory games. You could start by picturing the aisles in your supermarket, remember where everything is, visualise yourself in the shop, and remember what products are in each aisle. Or a good one to play with young grandchildren, is to collect several small objects from around the house, place them on a table, cover them with a cloth, try to remember what is there, and in turns add or take away items to test your alertness. Or simply spend some time with your memories. Look at old photograph albums and memorabilia and let your mind reflect on them and take you back to that place in time - it will repay you in positive emotions.

Puzzles

Some of us like crosswords, some logic puzzles or doing jigsaws. It really doesn't matter which kind you choose. Doing puzzles in your free time is a great way to activate your brain and keep it in good working condition. Do the puzzle for fun, and know you are exercising your brain at the same time.

Laughter

Laugh and maintain a positive attitude. Scientists tell us that laughter is good for our health; it releases endorphins and other powerful chemicals into our system. Laughter helps us reduce stress and can be like a 'quick charge' for our brain batteries. So make sure you laugh more.

Play

Take time to play. Play cards, videos, board games, computer games - it really doesn't matter what you play, just play. It's good for your spirits and it's good for your brain. Playing gives your brain a chance to think strategically and keep working.

Learn Something New

It is important to challenge our brain to learn new tasks. We capitalise on our brain's great potential when we put it to work learning new things, and it is one of the best ways to re-energise our brain.

Give your brain something new to concentrate on. Take up a new activity that will challenge it. Something you enjoy but have no knowledge of - learn a new language, take up tai chi or try learning a new word from the dictionary every day. Then test yourself at the end of the week.

Write

You can gain great value from writing for yourself. Whether it's writing in your journal, contemplative writing or penning the next best seller. Writing stimulates your brain and expands its capacity.

Exercise

We know that exercise is important for our physical health, and our brain is also part of that body. Increasing our blood flow through exercising brings more oxygen to the brain. Oxygen is fuel for the brain, which will help to improve your short-term memory loss and keep it active for many years to come.

This is a short and simple list, but an important one. I encourage you to apply at least one of these approaches every day - starting today.

Chapter Three

DIET AND NUTRITION

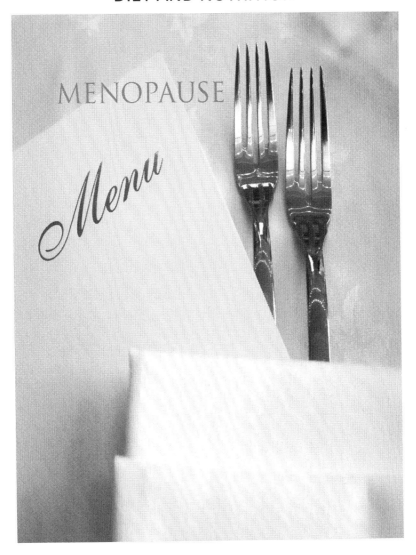

Managing Your Weight

About 90 percent of women will notice some weight gain during the menopause transition. On average they will gain 10-15lbs, and most of this weight will come on gradually at about a pound per year, unless you start to make some adjustments to your diet and exercise regime.

Why We Gain Weight

*Metabolism slows down.
*Fat cells contain oestrogen so your body holds on to them and converts more calories into fat for more oestrogen.
*Insulin Resistant – the body doesn't burn calories at the same rate as it used to; it stores them instead.
*Hormones start to distribute fat in the abdominal area rather than hips and thighs.

During the initial stages of this weight gain you may not make the connection with your waistband feeling a little tighter and menopause, but you will begin to start putting weight on around your middle instead of your hips and thighs. Also you will probably feel quite frustrated when you begin to notice these extra pounds, especially if you are eating and exercising exactly the same as you always were, but still can't seem to maintain your weight.
Don't blame yourself for this; it's not a case of you being greedy (unless you are of course!).
As you enter the early stages of menopause, maintaining weight becomes more difficult, and losing it even harder due to the fluctuation of your hormones.
Falling oestrogen levels seem to play their part in menopausal weight gain. As your ovaries begin producing less oestrogen, your body looks for other places to get this hormone. Fat cells can produce oestrogen so your body works harder to covert calories into fat to increase oestrogen levels – which is exactly the opposite of what we want to happen. Unfortunately, as we already know, fat cells don't burn calories the way muscle cells do, which causes you

to gain those extra pounds.

Progesterone - Lower levels of progesterone can cause water retention and bloating, which is one of the main symptoms of menopause, and although this doesn't actually result in weight gain, your clothes will probably feel a little tighter. The good news is water retention and bloating usually disappear within a few months.

Testosterone - Helps your body create lean muscle mass out of the calories you take in, and as muscle cells burn more calories than fat cells do, your metabolism is increased. Lower levels of testosterone result in loss of this muscle, leading to a lower metabolism and a slower rate for your body to burn calories.

Unhealthy Eating - Ready prepared meals, fast foods and take-a-ways all seem to fit nicely into our busy days; they are convenient and save us valuable time. But they could also be shortening your life. By being organised you could have a handful of healthy nutritious recipes to cook that are easy to prepare and won't take up too much of your time.
It is your responsibility to make sure the food your put into your body is beneficial and full of the nutrients you need to live a long and healthy life.

Lack of Exercise – If you don't prioritise exercise you won't do it. You will keep putting it off until tomorrow. It is very easy to fill your day with everyone else's demands, but you have to find the time to exercise, especially now. You should be doing at least 20-30 minutes of activities six to seven days a week. That doesn't mean you have to do intense training every day, just some sort of activity to strengthen and stretch your muscles and improve the strength of your heart - whether it's gardening, brisk walking or playing a round of golf - just do something.

Insulin Resistance

Insulin resistance is a condition in which the body produces insulin but does not use it properly.
The insulin hormone is the main factor in regulating the body's

metabolism. It is produced by the pancreas, which is a small organ that sits just behind the stomach. Once your food has been broken down into glucose, the simplest form of sugar that can be used by your cells, insulin starts to move the glucose into your cells to be used as energy, along with fat and protein.

Each cell in the body needs a continuous supply of glucose to satisfy its energy requirements; however, it cannot penetrate the outer membrane of a cell without the assistance of insulin. Insulin resistance happens when the cells essentially don't absorb the insulin.

When the cells become insulin resistant the pancreas has to make more insulin to try and do the same job. Insulin stimulates the body to convert glucose into fat, and then helps to block the fat from being released from the cells. In other words, it converts all a person's excess energy into fat and stores it away into fat cells. Once safely tucked away, insulin guards the fat by blocking it's release from the fat cells. We can become insulin resistant for a number of reasons, such as poor diet, lack of exercise or hormone imbalance, all of which are probably affecting you right now.

If you have developed insulin resistance during the menopause, not only will your body want to store the fat for as long as possible, but it will also recognise that it is a valuable supply of extra oestrogen and will be even more reluctant to let go of it. The excess of insulin will also affect your metabolism. For example if you eat 2000 calories a day, your body would normally burn 1400 and store the rest. However, if you are suffering from insulin resistance your body may only burn 600 calories and store 1400, which is a huge difference and one other reason why you gain weight.

Symptoms of Insulin Resistance
Exhaustion: Because cells aren't able to take up glucose and can't convert it into energy.
Drowsiness: Caused by blood sugar not being controlled.
Poor memory/foggy brain: The brain needs glycogen, if sugar in the blood is not converted into glycogen it will affect the function of the brain, including forgetfulness and foggy thinking.

So, with the effects of hormone imbalance and a slower metabolic rate, you are going to have to re-address your lifestyle. You will now need to exercise more - at least six days a week, revise your diet and be more aware of your portion sizes. You cannot expect to eat the same amount as you did when you were younger and stay the same size.

Why Your Waist Thickens in Menopause

When a woman's oestrogen levels drop during menopause, fat distribution and body shape also change. Hormonal changes alter the way your body breaks down and stores fat, which results in fat accumulating in your tummy and around your waist. The up side is you may notice your hips and thighs becoming slimmer.

Androgen hormones, including testosterone, are predominantly male hormones, but do occur in women in small quantities. Although androgen levels decrease during menopause, oestrogen levels drop at a higher rate, making androgen higher in ratio. This may cause women to gain fat where men do, such as the neck, chin and abdominal areas.

Studies also show that the hormone cortisol may have some effect on fat accumulating around your abdomen. Cortisol is released from the adrenal glands when the body is under stress. An elevation in cortisol levels has been shown to cause fat deposition in the abdominal area.

Genetics may play a part in your weight gain. If you have family members that gained weight around the abdomen, then it may affect you too.

Waist Circumference

Waist measurements provide information about the distribution of body fat. Carrying too much fat around your middle is associated with an increased risk of developing heart disease and diabetes,as well as greater risks of high cholesterol levels.

The fat that accumulates around your waist is a different type of fat than the rest of your body. This is known as 'visceral' fat, or intra-abdominal fat, and surrounds the internal organs, as well as the torso, and is usually a lot harder to lose than regular fat (subcutaneous) because it is more deeply embedded in the body's tissues. Therefore not only is this fat going to affect your weight, but also your overall health.

The liver, which is one of the most important organs in your body, is responsible for metabolising visceral fat and releasing it into the bloodstream as cholesterol. Although you need a certain amount of cholesterol in the body (to make hormones for one thing), the bad cholesterol can build up and block arteries, leading to strokes and heart attacks.

The good news is it responds well to a healthy diet and exercise.

Measure your waist without holding the tape too tightly (or loosely). As a rough guide your waist is the narrowest part of your torso, or approximately one inch above your belly button.

Waist circumference of over 31" (80cm) indicates slight health risk
Waist circumference of over 35" (90cm) indicates substantially increased health risks.

Waist/Hip Ratio

Waist to hip ratio is another check you can make to determine your overall health. It is a simple, yet accurate, method for determining your body fat pattern.

Research has shown that apple shapes are at a greater risk for developing a number of health-related problems, the most prominent being hypertension or high blood pressure, type II diabetes or non-insulin dependent diabetes, and hyperlipidaemia - (elevated levels of fat in the blood).

Abdominal fat cells tend to be larger than those located in other regions of the body. Relatively large fat cells are associated with insulin resistance, which means body cells will take up less glucose (sugar) from the blood, causing the blood sugar level to rise.

Measure your waist at its narrowest point and the hips at the widest point.

Now divide the waist circumference by the hip circumference.

0.80 or below = Low health risk
0.81-0.85 = Moderate health risk
0.85+ = High health risk

Quality of Food and Lifestyle

While it is true that hormone imbalance can cause weight gain, it is probably also a result of your lifestyle and the type of food you choose to eat. Especially the quick and easy meals readily available in most supermarkets, which are overloaded with salt, sugar, unhealthy fats and preservatives.

Even the quality of some unprepared food is questionable. Unfortunately for us, farmers can make more money by pumping their cattle full of hormones and growth enhancers and adding antibiotics to their feed. We get genetically modified food and crops sprayed with so many chemicals it's a wonder they don't glow in the dark, and chickens that never see the light of day.

The food business is a multi-billion pound industry and clever marketing can easily seduce us into believing that even a jam doughnut is as healthy as a fresh green salad.

Learn to read food labels and get into the habit of looking to see what is actually in that 'so called' healthy product. It won't take you long to figure out that all the fancy jargon on the front of the box, is probably quite contradictory to the nutritional facts on the label on the back. That healthy Muesli Bar you have been eating could actually be full of sugar and salt. Vitamin waters and health waters are another misnomer; some of these contain high levels of sugar and such small amounts of vitamins that they are of no nutritional benefit to you.

Fresh foods that are unprocessed and unrefined should be the mainstay of your diet and be eaten as close to their natural state as possible.

Buy organic if you can, so you know your fruit and vegetables have been grown in the healthiest of soils and have not been sprayed with any harmful chemicals.

Try visiting your local farmer's market and buy food that is in season so you get the best possible taste. Do we really need to eat raspberries in January that have been flown half way around to world and lost much of their flavour on the way?

Get to know your local butcher, ask where he gets his meat and if any growth hormones have been used. Again farmer's markets are good for this because the butcher will normally reared the cattle himself, and knows exactly where it was slaughtered and in what conditions, all resulting in a better quality meat.
If you are going to go to the trouble of improving your lifestyle to ensure a healthy, happy future, don't let the quality of your food let you down, otherwise your hard work could all be in vain, so make the time and the effort to source good quality products.

Lose the Weight
You don't have to resign yourself to the fact that weight gain is part of getting older. Staying healthy just requires a little more effort and will power, that's all. You need to invest in yourself to reap the rewards. So shift your focus and adjust your diet to incorporate what your body now needs and what it doesn't need. Keep active, both physically and mentally. By doing this you are giving yourself the best body you can and a pain free future to enjoy.

What Your Body Needs

The average daily calorie intake for a 50 year old woman is 1600, but this can vary between 1500 - 2000 depending on lifestyle and activity level.
If you are looking to lose weight you need to reduce your calorie intake by 500 per day to lose one pound in a week – 1lb of fat = 3,500 calories.

Your body can only use around 500-600 calories per meal so try to balance your calories during the day to prevent over-eating and to keep blood sugar levels stable.

Aim for :

- Breakfast 400 calories
- Lunch 400 calories
- Dinner 600 calories
- Snack 200 calories
- (2 snacks @ 100 calories each)

This example is based on 1600 calories per day; if your requirements are higher, then you can modify the formula to suit your lifestyle and caloric requirements. For example, if you're a big breakfast eater you may want to slightly adjust your calorie intake here and lower it for lunch if necessary, or if you prefer your main meal at lunch time rather than dinner adapt this to suit your needs.

BMR (Basal Metabolic Rate)

Work out how many calories you need by checking your BMR.

Basal Metabolic Rate (BMR) is the minimal caloric requirement needed to sustain life in a resting individual. This is the amount of energy your body would burn if you slept all day. It includes the body functions such as circulation, breathing, generating body heat, transmitting messages to the brain, cellular metabolism, and the production of body chemicals.

The easiest way to calculate your BMR is to use an online calculator. The result will provide an indication of how many calories your body needs each day to perform simple functions such as breathing and digesting food. You can also calculate your BMR based on how much physical activity you typically get, using a formula called the Harris Benedict Equation.

Alternatively, you can quickly determine you BMR using the basic 'rule of ten'. Multiply your weight by the number 10 and this is your BMR. For example if you weigh 150 pounds, you would have a BMR of 1500 calories - that means, when you are resting, your body needs 1,500 calories for natural processes such as blinking, breathing and swallowing.

Now add to that 20% of your BMR if you have a sedentary lifestyle; 30% if you are somewhat active; 40% if you are moderately active; or 50% if you are very active.

The number you get is how many calories you need to maintain your weight.
For example: If you're a somewhat active
150-pound woman, your BMR is 1500 calories a day, and your lifestyle activity level is 30% of that, - 1500 x 30% = 450 calories. So your daily total for maintaining your current weight is 1,950 calories. If you want to lose one pound per week, you simply need to cut or burn an extra 500 calories a day.

BMI (Body Mass Index)

This is a number calculated from your weight and height that correlates to the percentage of your total weight that comes from fat as opposed to muscle, bone or organ. The higher your BMI, the higher the percentage of fat in your body.
BMI under 20 = Underweight
Between 20-25 = Normal healthy weight
Over 25 = Overweight
Over 30 = Obese
There are many online calculators that will work out your BMI for you, or you can work it out manually by using the following formula:
Take your height in meters and multiply it by itself – e.g. 1.6 x 1.6 = 2.56
Divide your weight in kilograms by the answer above - so if your weight is 67 kilos,
67 ÷ 2.56 = 26.17
Your BMI is 26.17 - just putting you in the overweight category

Weight (lbs) & Height

Height	Low	Target	High
4ft 10"	100	115	131
4ft 11"	101	117	134
5ft	103	120	137
5ft 1"	105	122	140
5ft 2"	108	125	144
5ft 3"	111	128	148
5ft 4"	114	133	152
5ft 5"	117	136	156
5ft 6"	120	140	160
5ft 7"	123	143	164
5ft 8"	126	146	167
5ft 9"	129	150	170
5ft 10"	132	153	173
5ft 11"	135	156	176
6ft	138	159	179

Fig.4

Adjust Your Diet

It is important to eat food from all food groups to obtain the nutrients and minerals your body requires. During the menopausal transition you will need to slightly adjust your diet to optimise the health benefits of certain foods and the nutrients your body needs during this time, such as calcium, B Vitamins, Vitamins C, D, E, and K, magnesium and boron.

Portion Size
Portion size is important , most of us have gotten into the habit of eating far too much.
Over the years portion sizes have grown, along with our stomachs, and we now expect to see a certain amount of food on our plates, especially when eating out. We seem to equate good value with a plate over-laden with food, rather than good quality. Our mental attitude needs to change in this regard, and rather than feeling cheated by a smaller plate of food, we should see it as the correct amount we need. We do not need to overburden our digestive system and put a strain on our body by eating copious amounts of unnecessary food, which will only result in weight gain and a sluggish metabolism.

Try Using Smaller Plates
12 inches seems to be the size of the average dinner plate, try using a 9 inch size so that your smaller portions still look like a sizeable amount, but your calorie intake could be up to 25 percent less.

Food Groups

Foods groups will generally contain a combination of nutrients and are recommended in the following quantities in your menopause diet. Remember to eat slowly to allow your body to absorb the food as you consume it.

Breads/Cereals/Rice/Pasta=6 servings per day		
Examples	**One serving equals**	**That's about the size of**
Bread	1 oz. (1 small slice, ½ bagel, ½ bun)	A DVD
Cooked Grains	½ cup cooked oats, rice, pasta	Billiard ball
Dry Cereal	½ cup flakes, puffed rice, shredded wheat	Billiard ball

Fruits and vegetables =5-6 servings per day		
Examples	**One serving equals**	**That's about the size of**
Raw fruit	½ cup raw, canned, frozen fruit	Billiard ball
Dried fruit	¼ cup raisins, prunes, apricots	An egg
Juice	6 oz 100% fruit or vegetable juice	Hockey puck
Raw vegetables	1 cup leafy greens, baby carrots	Baseball
Cooked vegetables	½ cup cooked broccoli, potatoes	Billiard ball

Meat/Poultry/Fish/Beans=2 servings per day		
Examples	**One serving equals**	**That's about the size of**
Meat & Tofu	2-3 oz. cooked beef, poultry, fish, tofu	Deck of cards
Beans	½ cup cooked beans, split peas, legumes	Billiard ball
Nuts & Seeds	2 Tbsp. nuts, seeds, or nut butters	Ping pong ball
Dairy=2 Servings per day		
Examples	**One serving equals**	**That's about the size of**
Cheese	1 oz. or 1 thin slice of cheese	A pair of dice
Milk	1 cup milk, yogurt, soymilk	Baseball
Fats & Oils = small amounts		
Fat & Oil	1 tsp. butter, margarine, oil	One die

You may find it useful to mentally divide your plate into quarters:
¼ for meat/poultry/fish
¼ for potatoes/ rice/pasta (starchy foods)
½ for vegetables

Nutrients

Are what you get out of food, such as vitamins and minerals, and what is required by the body to live and function.
The different food groups supply these various nutrients in a form our bodies are able to absorb.

To simplify it, when you do your shopping, keep in mind that you need more carbohydrates than protein, meaning more fruit and vegetables than meat and fish, so there should be more of these types of food in your trolley.
The same applies when you cook your food. Most meals you prepare will have a combination of one or more of the food groups. What you need to try and achieve is the correct balance of these groups, and just by making a few simple changes you should be able to accomplish this. For example, a roast dinner - you need more vegetables than meat, or a spaghetti bolognese, more spaghetti than meat, and since this dish is short on vegetables you could add a few courgettes, carrots, or serve it with a side salad. Once you get into the habit of thinking about what food groups you need more or less of, you will be able to adjust most meals and get the balance correct. You could also try adjusting your meals slightly to make a healthier version of what you like.
For example try replacing refined sugars with natural honey for the added sweetness, swap butter for low fat spread, eat raw vegetables with your whole-wheat sandwich instead of crisps, use low fat meats like chicken and turkey and fill up on vegetables rather than potatoes, or try roasting the potatoes (with their skin on) along with the other vegetables in a small amount of olive oil and mixed herbs. Add a side salad to your meals to get a raw food fix, and instead of apple crumble and cream try cooked apples in a little honey and cinnamon, serve with low fat yoghurt and crunchy granola topping. Try replacing some of your tea and coffee each day with herbal drinks such as dandelion tea, which is a good liver cleanser.
Whatever you enjoy eating always try to prepare and cook it in the healthiest way possible and get into the habit of using nine inch plates to make sure you don't overeat.

*Stay away from white foods.
Flour, bread, rice, pasta, sugar, potatoes - if you eat white doughy foods you will look white, and doughy! (Hold that image in your head).
Opt for wholegrain varieties instead.

Nutrition Getting The Balance Right

Carbohydrates = 50% of daily diet
Fats = 30%-35% of daily diet
Protein = 15%-20% of daily diet
Fibre = 24gram

A healthy diet is a balanced diet. No food group should be eliminated.
Ensure your body gets all the nutrients it needs by eating food from each group every day.

Carbohydrates

(50% of daily diet – 230g approx.)

Carbohydrates are an important part of a healthy diet and are our main source of energy. They are found almost exclusively in plant foods such as fruits, vegetables, peas, beans and milk. Milk products are the only food derived from animals that contain carbs.
Carbohydrates have had a lot of bad press in the past, with some popular diets eliminating them totally, having us believe they are the root cause of all body fat and excess weight.
Unfortunately, the long-term effects of eating little or no carbs are still unknown and what is equally worrying is the inclusion of unhealthy foods in some of these diets.
Understand the difference between good carbs and bad carbs and choose them carefully.

The simplest way is to stay away from anything refined and eat food as close to its natural state as possible. Whole grains such as oats and pulses will break down quite slowly, keeping you fuller for longer, and blood glucose levels a lot more stable.

Whereas refined carbs found in white foods like pasta, potatoes, breads, and cakes, will not have much nutritional value and will be processed by your body quickly, leaving you feeling hungry again quite soon after eating them.

Most foods, however, do contain a mixture of both types of carbohydrates and it can be confusing to try and work out the 'good carb', 'bad carb' ratio.

The best way of doing this is to refer to their glycemic index (GI Index). This classifies carbs by how quickly and how high they boost blood sugar levels. The index ranks from 0 – 100 and the higher the G.I. the bigger the blood sugar rise. Foods with a score of 70 or higher are defined as having a high G.I. index and those with a score of 55 or below are low G.I., ensuring a slower and gentler change in blood sugar.

Do be aware though that you cannot use this G.I. index for a weight loss choice - for example a Snickers Bar has a G.I. of 41 making it a low G.I. food, but it's far from healthy.

Use it as a general guide to help you choose slow release energy foods, and where possible replace highly processed grains, cereals and sugars with minimally processed whole grains.

Glycaemic Index Tables
Table 1 –Low GI Foods (14 To 55)

Food	GI
Roasted and salted peanuts	14
Low-fat yoghurt with sweetener	14
Cherries	22
Grapefruit	25
Pearl barley	25
Red lentils	26
Whole milk	27
Dried apricots	31
Butter beans	31
Fettuccine pasta	32
Skimmed milk	32
Low-fat fruit yoghurt	33
Wholemeal spaghetti	37
Apples	38
Pears	38
Tomato soup, canned	38
Apple juice, unsweetened	40
White spaghetti	41

All Bran	42
Chick peas, canned	42
Peaches	42
Porridge made with water	42
Oranges	44
Macaroni	45
Green grapes	46
Orange juice	46
Peas	48
Baked beans in tomato sauce	48
Carrots, boiled	49
Milk chocolate	49
Kiwi fruit	52
Stoneground wholemeal bread	53
Crisps	54
Banana	55

Table 2
Medium GI Foods (56 to 69)

Food	GI
Muesli, non-toasted	56
Boiled potatoes	56
Sultanas	56
Pita bread	57
Basmati Rice	58
Honey	58
Digestive biscuit	59
Cheese and tomato pizza	60
Ice cream	61
New potatoes	62
Coca cola	63
Apricots, canned in syrup	64
Couscous	65
Rye bread	65
Pineapple, fresh	66
Cantaloupe melon	67
Croissant	67
Shredded wheat	67

Mars bar	68
Ryvita	69

You may include a few of the foods from Table 2 each day, but again limit portion sizes if you want to lose weight

Table 3
High GI Food (70+)

Food	GI
Mashed potatoes	70
White bread	70
Watermelon	72
Swede	72
Bagel	72
Bran flakes	74
Cheerios	74
French fries	75
Cocoa Pops	77
Jelly beans	80
Rice cakes	82
Rice Krispies	82
Cornflakes	84

Jacket potato	85
Puffed wheat	89
Baguette	95
Parsnips, boiled	97
White rice, steamed	98

Swap the foods from Table 3 for those with a low GI value, or eat them together with a low GI food. Having a jacket potato with baked beans, for example, will lower the GI value of that whole meal.

Try to consume low to medium carbohydrates. This will help to regulate your insulin and keep your blood sugar level balanced. The last thing you need in your life right now is your blood sugar going haywire at the same time as your hormones.
Eating low to medium G.I. foods can also help to reduce your mood swings and improve energy levels.

Good Carbs

- Main source of energy
- Good source of fibre
- Provides essential minerals and vitamins
- Improves mental concentration
- Strengthens muscle tissue
- Stabilises blood sugar levels

Bad Carbs

- Low in nutritional value
- High in calories
- Causes blood sugar levels to fluctuate
- Causes weight gain
- Causes lethargy
- Contributes towards heart disease

Fats

(30% - 35% of Daily Diet - 90g Approx.)

Fats are another nutrient that have received a bad reputation for causing weight gain, obesity and health problems, so you might be quite surprised to see that you required such a high amount. Fat is essential for survival and has a major role to play in the functioning of the body. The important thing is to distinguish the good fats from the bad fats

Good Fats
Polyunsaturated
Monounsaturated

Polyunsaturated Fats - There are two main types of polyunsaturated fat:
Omega 3
Omega 6
Both are essential fatty acids, meaning the body cannot make them and they must be provided by the diet.
Omega 3 helps the cell membranes to remain flexible and fluid - any deficiency can result in a wide variety of disorders including skin problems, easy bruising and swelling of joints.
It is also good for our brains, keeping the neurons and membranes flexible. As we age the membranes can stiffen, which can result in mood imbalances and problems with thinking and learning. Omega 3 can help restore these membranes, keeping them flexible and supple.

Omega 6 has many of the same benefits as omega 3, but has more effect on the skin and hair and can also help with menstrual disorders and symptoms.

Food Sources

Omega 3

- Oily fish (salmon, mackerel, halibut, herring)
- Broccoli
- Eggs
- Bread
- Peanuts
- Flaxseeds and oil
- Soy oil
- Walnuts
- Fruit juice

Omega 6

- Sunflower oil
- Sunflower seeds
- Peanuts
- Sesame seeds
- Evening primrose oil
- Chicken
- Olive oil

The ratio between omega 3 and omega 6 is important. Over recent years there seems to have been a dramatic increase of omega 6 and many people don't get enough omega 3. This is probably because it is more readily available in our everyday foods such as chicken, olive oil and sunflower oil.

An imbalance could result in chronic diseases such as heart disease, arthritis and diabetes as well as depression and accelerated ageing.

Omega 9

This is not technically an EFA because the body can provide a limited amount provided omega 3 and omega 6 are present. If your diet is low in these EFA's, then your body cannot produce omega 9 - which then becomes an essential fatty acid.

Main sources

- Olive oil
- Olives
- Avocados
- Peanuts
- Hazelnuts

Health Benefits

- Lowers cholesterol
- Reduces atherosclerosis (hardening of arteries)
- Reduces insulin resistance
- Improves immune function
- Protects against certain types of cancer

Monounsaturated Fats - Seem to be one of the healthiest fat choices, and studies show they can help lower the bad cholesterol without lowering the good. These fats have even more obvious beneficial effects when they are used to replace saturated fats in your diet.

Food Sources

- Avocados
- Almonds
- Hazelnuts
- Cashew nuts
- Sesame seeds
- Olive oil
- Grape seed oil
- Canola oil
- Peanut oil

Bad Fats
Saturated
Trans fats

Saturated fats come mainly from animal sources and some vegetable products.
These fats will increase cholesterol levels in the body, which can lead to hardening of the arteries and increase the risk of heart disease.
Try and keep them to a minimum of 20-30 grams per day - that's below 10 percent of your total daily calorie intake, and make sure you select low fat versions of these saturated fats where possible.

Food Sources
- Beef
- Veal
- Pork
- Ham
- Butter
- Milk
- Cheese
- Eggs
- Coconut oil
- Palm oil
- Vegetable shortening

Trans Fats
Can be even worse for you than saturated fats. Trans fats are made by heating liquid vegetable oil and adding hydrogen gas - a process called 'hydrogenation'. This procedure will extend the shelf life of a product and convert the oil into a solid, which also makes it easier for transportation. But while this may be extremely convenient and profitable for the manufacturers, it destroys all of the nutritional value the oil once had.
Trans fats confuse our body. This is not a natural fat, and if we don't have the enzymes to digest it properly it could raise the bad cholesterol in our body and lower the good, increasing your risk of heart disease.

Trans fats can be found in fried foods and baked goods. Make sure you keep these foods to a minimum, including fast foods and take-a-ways.

Look out for them in

- Margarines and spreads
- Pastries and pasties
- Biscuits
- Cereal bars
- Cakes and baking products
- Ice-creams, desserts and puddings

At present there is no safety level for trans fats; if you do eat them, eat no more than 4-5 grams per day.

Benefits of Good Fats

Helps absorb fat soluble vitamins A, D, E, and K.
Brain needs fat for development and protection.
Regulates production of hormones.
Promotes healthy cells.
Keeps skin cells plump and supple.
Helps regulate body temperature.
Protects our vital organs.
Carries flavour and adds taste and texture to food.

Dangers of Bad Fats

Increases cholesterol levels.
Clogs arteries.
Increases risk of heart disease.
Increases weight.
High blood pressure.

Eat More

- Olive oil
- Canola oil
- Sunflower oil
- Grape seed oil
- Salmon
- Mackerel
- Halibut

- Broccoli
- Eggs
- Avocados
- Chicken
- Flaxseeds
- Sunflower seeds
- Almonds
- Hazelnuts
- Peanuts
- Cashew nuts
- Sardines
- Tuna
- Trout
- Fruit juice

Eat Less

- Full fat dairy
- Beef
- Pork
- Veal
- Coconut oil
- Palm oil
- Pastries
- Baked goods
- Fried foods
- Biscuit, cakes and candy

Make The Switch To
Low fat dairy skimmed milk.
Grill, don't fry.
Eat more low fat meat - chicken and turkey.
Eat less beef, pork and veal.

Cholesterol

Our cholesterol levels are something else we have to pay attention to as we get older.

Cholesterol is not a fat, it's a waxy substance, and if you held it in your hand it would resemble the very fine scrapings of a whitish-yellow candle. Cholesterol forms part of the membrane that surrounds every cell in your body.

The liver makes cholesterol from carbohydrates, fats and protein. It is transported via the blood-stream to every part of your body, where it is used in various ways - such as protecting cell membranes, helping nerve cells to send messages, enabling the gall bladder to make bile, absorbing fat soluble vitamins, and as we know, it is used to make hormones such as oestrogen, progesterone and testosterone.

When our body makes cholesterol it is normally very well controlled, so that if we eat too much cholesterol in our diet, we make less in our body. But an excessive intake of saturated fats can significantly raise the blood cholesterol level, which can make its way into blood vessels, stick to the walls and form deposits that eventually block the flow of blood, causing clogging and hardening of the arteries.

Having a high level of cholesterol in the blood doesn't make you feel ill or different in anyway, and you may have absolutely no warning that a stroke or heart attack is going to happen until it actually begins.

Good cholesterol (HDL) is responsible for taking excess cholesterol away from your arteries to the liver to be eliminated from the body. Bad cholesterol (LDL) takes the cholesterol from your liver to the body tissues and can build up in the walls of the blood vessels, causing them to narrow.

One of the biggest misconceptions people have is that food is packed with cholesterol. In fact very little cholesterol is found in food, the main culprits are eggs, offal and shell fish.

What is important is the type of fat in the food you choose, especially the saturated fat. Once inside the body the liver turns this fat into cholesterol.

Protein

(15%-20% of daily diet - 44g approx.)

Protein is essential for growth, development and to build healthy bones. It provides the body with energy and is necessary for the manufacture of hormones, anti-bodies, enzymes and tissues. It forms part of the structure of every cell in your body including muscles, skin, hair and nails. So during menopause it is essential to include the right amount of protein in your diet.

Your body cannot store protein so it must be supplied on a daily basis from the foods you eat.

Some foods are known as 'complete proteins' and contain all the essential amino acids (which are the building blocks for all proteins). Proteins obtained from animals are good sources as the animal has already processed the vegetable matter for us. Proteins obtained from plant sources are incomplete, meaning they are deficient in one or more amino acids. So in order to get all the essential amino acids from plants, you would need to combine different plant sources – which isn't that difficult and is probably part of your diet already, for example beans on toast or pasta with a cheese sauce.

However, eating too much protein can put a strain on the kidneys and may increase calcium loss from the bones.

As your body digests protein, it releases acids into the blood stream that the body neutralises by drawing calcium from the bones. So although it is important to eat protein on a daily basis, make sure you don't eat too much.

Good Sources of Protein Include

- Salmon
- Cod
- Halibut
- Trout
- Sea bass
- Tuna (canned in water)
- Chicken
- Turkey
- Lean steak
- Lean beef

- Milk
- Yoghurt
- Cottage cheese
- Ricotta
- Mozzarella
- Cheddar cheese
- Parmesan
- Feta
- (Choose low fat dairy products)
- Lima beans
- Lentils and most beans
- Almonds
- Peanuts
- Cashews
- Sunflower seeds
- Pumpkin seeds
- Flaxseeds
- Fermented tofu

Good For
Muscle development.
Builds and repairs tissues.
Promotes hair and nail growth.

Bad Because
Too much protein leads to acidity.
Calcium is drawn from bones to balance this effect.

Choosing The Right Soy

We are encouraged to eat soy for its complete protein content, low fat, phyto-oestrogens and other nutritional benefits. But it is important to choose the right soy products or there may be no benefit to you at all.

Soy foods are divided into two groups: fermented soy and non-fermented soy.

Fermented soy includes: miso, tempeh, soy sauce and natto.

Non-fermented soy includes: tofu, soymilk, yoghurts, and cheese.

Fermented soy reigns supreme and is the one most beneficial for you during menopause.

What you may not know about soy is it is one of the most genetically modified crops on the planet, and is used for both human consumption and animal feed. Unfortunately, we don't know what the long-term risks are, as scientists only have around 10 years of data on the GM crop.
Soybeans are also high in something called phytic acid or phytates. This is an organic acid present in the bran or hull of all seeds, but is highest in the soybean, and it blocks the uptake of essential minerals such as calcium, magnesium, iron and especially zinc in the intestinal tract, and is very difficult to digest. Furthermore, it is highly resistant to soaking and cooking, even long, slow cooking will not reduce the phytic acid in the soybean as it does in all other beans. Only a long period of fermentation will significantly reduce the phytate content. Thus, fermented products such as tempeh and miso provide nourishment that is easily assimilated, but the nutritional value of unfermented soy products such as tofu and bean curd, both high in phytates is questionable.

Fermented soy is the main soy consumed in Japan albeit in relatively small amounts, where countless studies have linked soy intake to longevity and very low cancer and heart disease rates, as well as far fewer menopausal symptoms.

The safest way to eat soy is whole, organic and fermented.

If you are using unfermented soy food products such as tofu, soymilk, cheese, yoghurts and edamame, it is best to limit your intake to just a few servings a week. Some experts believe you should avoid all unfermented soy products.

Natural toxins in unfermented soy block the enzyme trypsin that help you digest protein and the high levels of phytic acid block your ability to absorb calcium magnesium, copper, iron and zinc.

Fermented Soy Products

Miso - Richly salted, fermented paste, made from soybeans alone or mixed with grains such as rice, barley and wheat. Good for making soups, stock and broth. Works well with noodles and vegetables.

Shoya - (Soy Sauce) Originally a by-product of miso. This brown liquid is used as seasoning in many Asian dishes.

Tamari - (Soy Sauce) Also a by-product of miso but without added grains.

Tempeh - Soybeans combined with rice or millet and a mould culture for 24 hours. It's a meat like cake that can be grilled or added to main dishes.

Natto - Is a sticky paste mixture - not that popular with Europeans due to its pungent smell. Can be added to vegetable dishes or as a rice topping.

Fermented Tofu - Is made from cooked and pureed soybeans and then fermented to make a creamy food resembling soft cheese which can be used in a variety of dishes.

Fermented Soymilk - Is made from soymilk that has been fermented by pro-biotic bacteria.

Fibre

(24g per day)

There are two main types of fibre:
Insoluble
Soluble

Fibre is technically a carbohydrate, the difference is you can't digest it.

Coming from the part of the plant that is resistant to the body's digestive enzymes, it cannot be broken down into sugar molecules nor absorbed by the body. Most plants contain a mixture of both types of fibre.

Insoluble fibre - is the tough fibrous part of the plant and you will find it in whole-wheat bread, pasta, breakfast cereals, wholegrain rice.Small amounts are found in fruit and vegetables.

It absorbs water, will help you to feel full after eating and stimulates your intestinal walls to move solid materials, bulk faeces and make them softer.

Soluble fibre - is found mostly in pulses such as beans and lentils, oats, fruit and vegetables. It seems to lower the amount of cholesterol circulating in your blood and may offer some protection against heart disease. Soluble fibre can also make you feel full without adding calories.

Fibre is not a nutrient; it contains no calories or vitamins but is vital to good health. You will find it in all plant foods, but there is absolutely no fibre in meat, fish, poultry, milk, milk products or eggs.

Phyto-Oestrogens

Certain foods contain hormone-like components called phyto-oestrogens. They have a similar structure to the hormone oestrogen and can bind to oestrogen receptors throughout the body, mimicking the effects of oestrogen. It is thought they may help to alleviate some symptoms during menopause such as hot flushes and vaginal dryness.

There are three main groups of phyto-oestrogens:

Isoflavones
Found in soybeans, lentils, chickpeas, pinto beans, haricot beans, peanuts.

Coumestans
Found in sprouting beans, alfalfa, mung bean sprouts, soybean sprouts.

Lignans
Found in flaxseeds, rye bran, whole wheat, barley, sesame seeds, pumpkin seeds, fruit and vegetables.

Phyto-oestrogens are found in many fresh foods so you will probably be eating them already anyway. Or a simple way to increase your intake is to add one tablespoon of ground flaxseed to your food, add it to yoghurts, sprinkle it on salads or mix into your main meal. Freshly ground flaxseed contains much greater concentrations of lignans, protein and fibre.

*Note – flaxseeds must be ground to get their full nutritional value - do not eat them whole.

Foods Rich In Phyto-Oestrogens

Apples	Sunflower seeds	Navy beans	Soy
Alfalfa sprouts	Cherries	Red beans	Millet
Celery	Olives	Split Peas	Barley
Parsley	Pears	Ginger	Flaxseeds
Beets	Plums	Cloves	Lentils
Bok choy	Prunes	Oregano	Kidney beans
Broccoli	Barley	Sage	Lima beans
Cauliflower	Oats	Thyme	Rye
Mushrooms	Brown rice	Turmeric	Chick peas
Brussel sprouts	Wheat germs	Seaweeds	Fennel
Squash	Pumpkin seeds	Black eye peas	Mung beans

If you are oestrogen dominant then you may want to keep these foods to a minimum.

Menopause Super Foods

There are many foods that crop up time and again that are extremely beneficial for us during menopause, such as broccoli which is rich in calcium phyto-oestrogens, vitamin C, potassium and fibre, or flaxseeds which are rich in omega 3, phyto-oestrogens and protein. All super foods are rich in nutrients, with high levels of antioxidants that help the body fight cell damage from free radicals and protect us against diseases such as cancer, strokes and heart disease.
Nutrient rich foods provide many health benefits and super foods are thought to contain higher concentrations of these nutrients.

These menopause super foods are especially rich in the nutrients your body needs during this time:

Dandelion Greens
Are low in calories and high in vitamins, especially vitamin A and C as well as calcium, potassium and foliate. They can be used in salads or sautéed with garlic and pepper.
Dandelion tea is also beneficial for cleansing the liver.

Grapefruits
Are high in nutrients, each 1 cup serving gives more than 100 percent of daily recommended vitamin C which helps to neutralise free radicals.

Tempeh
Made from fermented soybeans, rich in protein and may ease menopause symptoms because of the phytochemicals it contains. Use in soups, salads and sandwiches.

Seaweed
Sea vegetables are rich in vitamins and minerals. Kelp is an excellent source of iodine and has 10 times more calcium than milk. Nori, the seaweed wrapped around sushi contains protein, calcium, magnesium, iron, potassium and more vitamin A than carrots. Try putting kelp into a shaker and use it to replace salt, or crumble nori sheets and sprinkle on salads.

Avocados
People shy away from avocados because of their high fat content. But it is good fat that your body needs, and they also contain nearly 20 different vitamins, minerals and phytonutrients.

Prunes
Are high in antioxidants and have more potassium than bananas. Potassium helps keep our blood pressure in check.

Beets
Are a great source of fibre, vitamin C and iron. Try adding to salads or roasting them with other vegetables.

Pumpkin
High in fibre and beta-carotene, an antioxidant that can help improve immune function and reduce risks of cancer and heart disease. Try marinating in olive oil and balsamic vinegar then roasting.

Wheatgrass
Is high in chlorophyll, which has many benefits including neutralising toxins, helps to purify the liver, improves blood sugar problems, improves digestion and can increase the function of the heart and lungs. To get the full benefit of chlorophyll it must be from a living plant.
Wheatgrass is a rich source of calcium, iron, magnesium and potassium, has more vitamin C than oranges and twice the vitamin A of carrots and is exceptionally rich in vitamins E, K and B complex.

Pomegranates
Are high in vitamin K, potassium and magnesium and, also a good source of Vitamin E and B6. Use in fruit salads, green salads. The juice provides a concentrated source of antioxidants and nutrients.

Watercress
Is high in vitamins A, C and K and is a good source of potassium, magnesium and calcium. Use in stir fries, salads, soups and sandwiches.

FSA
Flaxseeds
Sunflower seeds
Almonds
Mix equal parts together, put in grinder or use in a mill.
Suitable to use on all foods and has a plethora of nutritional benefits.

Anti-Oxidants and Free Radicals

Anti-oxidants help to protect the body from harmful free radicals. When oxygen is metabolised in our body it creates free radicals, which steal electrons from other molecules causing damage to our cells.
Free radicals are normally present in our body in small numbers which we actually need for activating enzymes, helping to destroy viruses and bacteria and producing vital hormones.
Under normal circumstances our body can keep them in check. However, if there is excessive free radical formation, damage to cells and tissues can occur. Many different factors can lead to an excess of free radicals such as smoking, sun exposure, pollution and lack of exercise. Diet can also contribute to their formation, particularly a diet high in fat, because oxidation occurs more readily in fat molecules than it does in carbohydrate or protein molecules.
Cooking with fats at high temperatures, in particular frying foods in oil, can produce large numbers of free radicals.
Antioxidants are beneficial because they neutralise free radicals by giving them a free electron to make them stable.

There are many types of anti-oxidants available from the food we eat and they are included in many of the lists earlier in this chapter, so you shouldn't have too much of a problem including them in your daily diet. Look out for them in:

Foods High In Anti-Oxidants

Onions	Lentils	Leeks
Spinach	Garlic	Seeds
Seafood	Parsley	Lean meat
Mangoes	Broccoli	Berries
Cabbage	Apricots	Soybeans
Green tea	Red wine	Tomatoes
Whole Grains	Vegetable oils	Beets

Important Vitamins and Minerals During Menopause

Try to get as many of your vitamins and minerals in their natural form from food, which is thought to be the most beneficial way for the body to process them. Only use supplements when you are having difficulty reaching your recommended daily requirements.

Don't succumb to thinking that more is better by popping a vitamin pill as added insurance to better health. You are trying to balance your body by giving it what it needs, any surplus will be excreted, or certain vitamins could possibly be stored and become toxic to the body.

Vitamin A - (RDA 700mcg) – Fat Soluble
A fat soluble vitamin which plays an important role in vision, bone growth, skin repair and may help maintain healthy vaginal tissue. Vitamin A can come from animal sources including liver, eggs and whole milk and is absorbed in the form of retinol. Vitamin A found in colourful fruits and vegetables is a carotenoid, also known as pro-vitamin A.

Common carotenoids found in foods from plants are beta-carotene and alpha carotene.

Some foods such as skimmed dairy will be fortified with vitamin A to replace the amount lost when the fat is removed.

Vitamin B Complex
The B-complex vitamins are actually a group of eight vitamins, which include:

Thiamin – B1 RDA – 1.5mg
Riboflavin – B2 1.7mg
Niacin – B3 15-20mg
Pantothenic acid – B5 10mg
Pyridoxine – B6 1.5mg
Biotin – B7 300mcg
Cyanocobalamin – B12 4-6mcg
Folic Acid 400mcg

B vitamins are essential for growth and development.
In particular during menopause, B3 helps support mental clarity and memory, B5 is essential for proper brain function and B6 helps with hormone production.
Deficiency of certain B vitamins can cause anaemia, tiredness, depression, hair loss and muscle cramps. Good sources of B3 are liver, fish, chicken, lean red meat, nuts and whole grains. B5 is

found in almost all foods. The richest sources of vitamin B6 are found in fish, beef, liver and other organ meats, potatoes, other starchy vegetables, and fruit (other than citrus).

Some doctors and nutritionists suggest taking the B-complex vitamins as a group for overall good health. However, most agree that the best way to get our B vitamins is naturally - through the foods we eat, and because we don't need them in large amounts, it shouldn't be difficult to obtain them from a healthy diet.

Vitamin C - (RDA 2,000mg)
An anti-oxidant that blocks some of the damage caused by free radicals. This vitamin is required for growth and repair of tissues, essential for healing of wounds, repair and maintenance of cartilage, bones and teeth and may help with hot flushes and moods swings.

The body does not make vitamin C, nor does it store it, so it is important to include it in your daily diet. All fruits and vegetables contain some amount of vitamin C. The highest sources come from green peppers, citrus fruits and juices, strawberries, tomatoes, broccoli, leafy green vegetables, papaya, mango, watermelon, Brussel sprouts and cabbage.

Vitamin E - (RDA 500mg – 250mg x twice a day) - fat soluble.
An anti-oxidant that helps reduce the damage caused by toxic chemicals. Vitamin E helps the body to use vitamin K and some studies have found it can lower the risks of heart disease and reduce the risks of strokes in post-menopausal women. Some women find it helps relieve hot flushes, vaginal dryness and improves health of skin and nails.

The richest source of vitamin E is wheat germ. Other foods with significant high amounts are liver, eggs, nuts (almonds, hazelnuts & walnuts), sunflower seeds, dark green leafy vegetables, avocados and asparagus.

Vitamin D (RDA 15mcg) - fat soluble
Essential for the absorption of calcium. The main source of vitamin

D is from the sunlight, which your body then converts into Vitamin D - 15 minutes a day will fulfill your daily requirement. Very few foods contain vitamin D - mackerel, eggs, fortified dairy products and some breakfast cereals.

Calcium (RDA 1500mg)
In addition to strengthening the bones, calcium is extremely important for the contraction of muscles, including the heart muscle. Low or high levels of calcium can quickly lead to disturbances in the cardiac rhythm. All dark green vegetables are a good source of calcium except spinach which blocks calcium absorption; broccoli is particularly high in calcium.

Magnesium (RDA 400mg)
Magnesium is a mineral that helps bones absorb calcium. It has a calming effect and can ease symptoms like anxiety, mood swings and insomnia. It helps to lower blood cholesterol and relax muscles. Good sources of magnesium can be found in almonds, cashew nuts, kale, kelp and wheat bran. If you feel you need to take magnesium supplements, make sure you use magnesium citrate, as this is most easily absorbed by the body and it should be taken with food. Be aware that an excess of magnesium can cause nausea and diarrhoea; try lowering the dose if this occurs.

Boron (RDA 3.0mg)
This mineral helps raise levels of oestrogen and decreases the amount of calcium excreted in urine. Boron can be found in apples, pears, dark green leafy vegetables, honey, almonds, raisins, figs, peaches, strawberries and sesame seeds.

Water

We all know by now that we should be drinking six to eight 8 ounce glasses of water a day to stay hydrated.

The human body is composed of approximately 70 percent water. Water is contained in the cells of our bodies, in the arteries and veins and all the spaces in between.

The body's water supply is used in nearly every bodily process. The water distributes nutrients and hormones, maintains body temperature and removes waste products.

So there really is no question that we need water to survive. The 8 glass theory was worked out as an average of what you would need to replace water lost during the day; this will vary slightly if you are more active than the average person or live in a hot climate, where you lose more water through perspiration. Adjust the levels to suit your lifestyle and remember your body gets fluids not only from the water you drink but also from the food you eat, especially fruit and vegetables.

Drink water to fulfil your requirements. Don't drink it excessively thinking it to be more beneficial. Researchers found that as you drink more water, your ability to filter toxins out of the blood actually goes down. They found no evidence that drinking a lot of water improves your skin or any other organ.

Too much water and not enough salt in your diet can be fatal.

Most people know that dehydration can result in serious health consequences – what a lot of people don't realise is that too much water can also be dangerous, even deadly.

Water intoxication, or 'hyponatraemia' happens when the body's balance of salt and water become quickly diluted. If you force large amounts of water into your system over a short period of time, your kidneys will struggle to eliminate enough water from your system to keep the overall amount at a safe level. In an effort to make an equal balance of salt and water, water will begin to seep into your cells from your blood, causing the cells to swell. If this swelling occurs in your brain, the bones that make up your hard skull can hardly move to accommodate it. The result is increased pressure and your brain gets squeezed, resulting in headaches, impaired breathing and the

most serious of all – death.
Be sensible, maintain your daily quota of water intake and drink if you are thirsty. Leave the rest up to your body. It's more than capable of looking after you.

Salt

(RDA 6g per day or 1 teaspoon)

Salt is an essential nutrient that we cannot live without. It is a vital component of all human body fluids including blood, sweat and the very tears we cry.
We each have about a cupful of salt in our body at any one time and it is doing a vital job in keeping us alive.
One of its primary roles is maintaining a proper balance of fluids in the body to regulate the movement of fluids into and out of our cells.

Our body cannot make salt so we must get it from our diet, which isn't that difficult because over 75 percent of our daily intake comes from the foods we eat, such as ham, soups, breads, cereals, tinned food and ready meals.

Electrolytes
Sodium, chloride and potassium are the 3 major electrolytes. Electrolytes control the fluids going in and out of the body tissues and cells.

Sodium - Potassium Balance
Our cells require an intricate balance of sodium and potassium for fluid balance. The potassium resides inside our cells while the sodium bathes the outside and between cells.
When we have the correct balance, our nerves and muscles are

strong. When the balance is off, muscles become weak, we lack muscle tone, and our reflexes become poor.

Grains, fruit and vegetables all have good potassium content. Avoid coffee, alcohol and refined sugars - which deplete potassium.

Healthy Salt Substitute

The problem with common table salt is it's a highly refined version of naturally occurring salt. Natural salt, whether sea salt or rock salt, contains over 60 trace minerals, including sodium chloride, iodine and potassium. The salt you find in supermarkets or restaurants and in processed foods has normally been stripped of its complex combination of trace minerals. It is refined down to sodium chloride and then conditioned with anti-caking chemicals, potassium and iodine. Dextrose (sugar) is added to stabilise the iodine.

This is the type of salt that has been linked to so many modern health problems. Like all other highly processed foods and substances, refined salt is denatured and lacking all the benefits of its whole food version.

Be careful when buying salt. Just because it carries the 'natural' label doesn't mean it is a whole food. It may still be refined or pure white, while natural salt is slightly grey and may even have a pinkish hue. Celtic sea salt, Dead Sea salt and Himalayan salt are good whole food varieties.

Remember salt is beneficial, and we need it in our diet, but too much salt can be detrimental to our health, especially during menopause, as it is one of the things that leaches calcium from our bones.

A craving for salt may be a craving for the natural minerals in unrefined salt. Minerals are the basis for the formation of vitamins, enzymes and proteins and are essential for healthy bodily function. One of the critical minerals is potassium; our cells require an intricate balance of sodium and potassium.

Eat a wide range of mineral rich foods such as seaweeds, miso, tamari, beets, celery, spinach, kale and parsley.

Cut out refined salt and replace with the whole food variety or try using Gomasio.

Gomasio

A traditional Japanese condiment made from toasted sesame seeds and sea salt.

Using this blend of sesame and salt instead of table salt is a great way to reduce sodium in the diet as well as strengthen digestion. Sesame seeds mixed with salt or seaweed make a powerful anti-acid that alkalises the blood and brings the PH back into balance. Traditional Gomasio is a simple 5:1 ratio of toasted sesame seeds to sea salt, crushed with a mortar and pestle.

You can also buy ready to use seaweed Gomasio that includes dulse, nori and Kombu seaweeds along with the sesame and salt, which is also a nourishing way to re-mineralise and alkalise your body while cutting back on sodium. It makes a satisfying topping for salads, soups, pastas or any foods you would normally add salt to at the table.

Recipe

¼ cup sesame seeds
1 teaspoon dulse flakes
1 teaspoon nettle leaf (cleanses body of excess salt)
½ teaspoon sea salt (optional)

Toast sesame seeds over medium heat until slightly golden, cool seeds and mix with dulse flakes and nettle leaf in blender, grinder or mortar and pestle.

Grind coarsely. If dulse and nettle leaf are whole, grind these into flakes first.

Mix together and add optional salt if desired.
Store in jar or large shaker. Can also be used in a spice mill. Keep in fridge to maintain freshness.

Try mixing with other edible seaweeds like nori, kombu and kelp granules, or a blend of all seaweeds will work well.

Recipe 2 (salt free Gomasio)
1 part nettle leaf
1 part celery seeds
1 part sesame seeds
½ part milk thistle seeds
½ part fennel seeds
½ part dry onion or garlic

Mix together and place in grinder to use.
Variations: Try some dry citrus rind, pepper or mustard seeds.

Acid/Alkaline Balance

Our body is designed to be slightly alkaline at a PH of 7.36 and it will do anything it has to in order to maintain this balance.

If the body becomes acidic it calls upon the stores of alkaline buffers which it draws upon to neutralise the acids we ingest or create through bodily processes.

Most of us tend to eat and drink more acidic foods than we should, and anything that makes the blood acidic will leach calcium from the bones to neutralise the acids. Animal protein and some dairy products (which are also high in protein) will actually leach more calcium than gets absorbed due to their high levels of acidity in the body, which is not good for the menopausal woman.

Diet, stress, emotions and no exercise also contribute to increased acidity in our body
PH is the abbreviation for 'Power of Hydrogen' and measures the acidity and alkalinity of a solution.

The scale goes from 0 - 14 with 7 being neutral

14 = maximum alkalinity and 0 = maximum acidity

Normal blood PH of a human is 7.36 making it slightly alkaline. Anything above is considered alkaline and anything below is considered acidic.

Try to balance your diet with 70 – 80 percent of it being alkaline foods.

A diet rich in vegetables will help keep your body's alkaline/acid balance at the right levels.

Never eat a meal that consists solely of acidic foods.

The amount of alkaline foods should always be greater than acidifying foods.

Do not consume a diet of alkaline foods only for more than 2 weeks.

Drink ironised water; it is very alkaline and will dissolve any accumulation of acid waste.

Swap some of your daily drinking water and cooking water for ironised water to help restore the balance.

Acid in the stomach often declines with age. It is important to remember that stomach acid is vital for digestion and proper absorption of calcium. Apple cider vinegar can create an acidic stomach environment which aids the absorption of calcium.

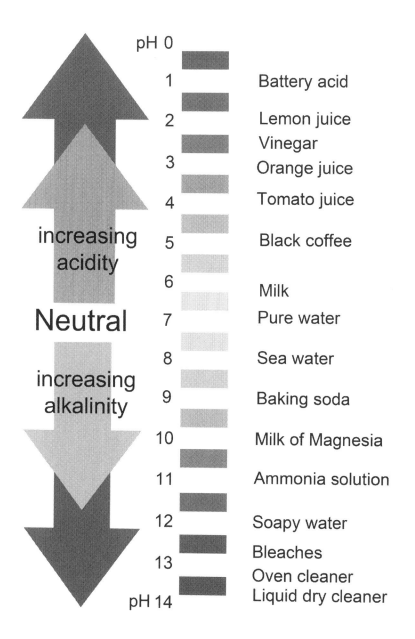

pH 0

1 Battery acid

2 Lemon juice
   Vinegar
3 Orange juice

4 Tomato juice

increasing
acidity   5 Black coffee

6
   Milk

Neutral 7 Pure water

8 Sea water

increasing
alkalinity 9 Baking soda

10 Milk of Magnesia

11 Ammonia solution

12 Soapy water

13 Bleaches
    Oven cleaner
pH 14 Liquid dry cleaner

Acidic Foods

- Sugar
- Trans Fats
- Dairy
- Refined Carbs
- Alcohol
- Fizzy drinks
- Pizza
- French fries
- Biscuits
- Crisps
- Bread
- Caffeine
- Fatty meats
- Ice-cream
- Milky drinks
- Cream

Alkaline Foods

- Fresh Vegetables
- Salads
- Leafy greens
- Omega 3 Oils
- Nuts
- Seeds
- Whole grains

*More information on Acid-Alkaline diets can be found at www.balance-ph-diet.com

The Great Dairy Debate

This topic really goes beyond the realms of this book and is quite a controversial subject.

But, we will touch on it lightly and you can come to your own conclusion about what's right for you.

In a 12 year study at Harvard University, 78,000 women who got most of their calcium from dairy products actually broke more bones than women who rarely drank milk, and a similar study in Australia showed that higher dairy consumption was associated with increased fracture risk.

We have already mentioned that the source of all calcium is from the soil, or the sea (in the form of seashells and coral). Calcium is technically a metal found mostly in rocks. Soils containing those rocks absorb calcium from them, which is in turn absorbed by the plants grown in that soil. Even cows get their calcium from plants. To date, there is no scientific evidence to prove that dairy products prevent bone disorders and osteoporosis. In fact research shows that countries with the highest rate of osteoporosis, including the USA, Finland and Sweden, consume the most dairy.

In order for calcium to be absorbed and used by the body there must be an equal quantity of magnesium and sufficient amounts of vitamin D. Magnesium and vitamin D aid the absorption of calcium into the bones, and cow's milk by itself does not have enough of either to support its calcium - which is why you will often see milk fortified with Vitamin D. In reality, only about twenty-five percent of dairy calcium from milk can be absorbed.

This can cause excessive calcium to accumulate in the body, which in turn can lead to the development of harmful calcium deposits in our joints, cause kidney stones to develop, and plaque to build-up in the arteries of the heart; it can also be a contributing factor for arthritis and gout.

Milk and dairy products are also high in protein, which can make the blood acidic. When this happens the body will try and re-balance itself by using calcium which it will leach from the bones.

The only reason people still believe that cow's milk is the best, and perhaps even the sole source of calcium for human beings is because of the promotional efforts carried out by the dairy industry.

Calcium is available from so many other sources such as: kale, broccoli, almonds, sardines and canned salmon with bones, oranges, sweet potatoes and sesame seeds to name but a few, and because there is an equal balance of magnesium in these foods they lend themselves to proper calcium assimilation in the body.

Remember, even if milk shows a higher calcium level content, it will not be absorbed as well by the body due to its lack of magnesium and vitamin D.

Maybe if we ate what cows eat - mainly plants, then we could get all the calcium we need.

Drink milk if you enjoy it but don't be seduced by the advertising jargon.

Love Your Liver

As we know oestrogen, progesterone, testosterone and the stress hormone cortisol are all steroid hormones, originally made from cholesterol, which is produced in the liver. The liver is also responsible for eliminating excess hormones and trying to keep the balance right in your body. So it is important to support your liver as much as you can, especially during this stage of your life.

The liver is not only responsible for making and balancing our hormones, it is also our primary detoxification organ and manufacturing plant. This organ has to deal with thousands of types of toxins all day, such as car fumes, cigarette smoke, cosmetic chemicals, and agricultural chemicals just to name a few. It deals with these toxins by either getting rid of them directly via the gall bladder, in the bile it manufacturers, or through the digestive track as it converts them into safer compounds, like the conversion of ammonia (which is a by-product formed by the breakdown of proteins in the body) into urea, which is a waste compound that the body then excretes in urine.

This efficient process of toxins can protect you from a variety of degenerative diseases including heart disease, diabetes and arthritis.

What You Eat Can Affect Your Liver

If you consume a lot of processed foods the additives can eventually affect the liver

An impaired liver will not be able to process food or detoxify substances as rapidly or as completely as a healthy liver, and if the liver isn't producing enough bile it cannot adequately digest fats. This can result in more toxic substances circulating in the body. These toxins can build up, and over time will be stored in the fatty tissues in the body as well as in the cells of the brain and central nervous system. These stored toxins may then be slowly released, contributing to many chronic illnesses.

In terms of self-help the best thing you can do is change your diet. Eat plenty of fresh vegetables and fruits, organic if possible, so you know your liver doesn't have to process any chemicals. Lemons are particularly good for the liver as they contain hydrochloric acid, needed for protein digestion. Try a glass of warm water with freshly squeezed lemon juice first thing every morning.

Steam foods and eat little, light and early in the day. This means less work for the liver. Avoid processed foods, fatty foods, alcohol, margarine and coffee; all of these substances add toxins to the body, making it more difficult to cleanse the liver.

Walk after meals and consider taking herbal supplements that are valuable to the liver and detoxification. Milk Thistle, liquorice, apple cider vinegar and dandelion tea are all particularly good for this.

Top 10 Foods for Looking After Your Liver

1. **Garlic** - Contains sulphur which helps the liver to detoxify a wide range of poisonous compounds including medications, alcohol and pesticides. Other sulphur containing foods include onions and egg yolks.

2. **Oat Bran** - Good source of water-soluble fibre. Oat bran aids in the elimination of bile and cholesterol that the liver produces when you eat fatty foods and oils.

3. **Brussel Sprouts** - Contain a large amount of vitamin K. which helps support the liver. People with liver problems are often deficient in this vitamin. Other sources include alfalfa sprouts, spinach, broccoli and kale.

4. **Artichokes** - Have long been used in treating liver disorders. The active ingredient in this cleansing food is caffeoylquinic acid, which protects and helps regenerate the liver.

5. **Organic Chicken** - Limited amounts of lean high protein foods such as organic chicken, fish or fermented tofu maintain growth and development of all your body tissues and prevent fatty build up in the liver.

6. **Turmeric** - This common spice contains the pigment curcumin which has traditionally been used in Ayurvedic medicine to treat liver and gallbladder disorders.

7. **Dandelion** - Dandelion leaves contain more nutrients than many other vegetables. This herb, which you will find as part of many green salad mixes, enhances the flow of bile, helping to improve the liver function. Dandelion tea is also beneficial and can be found in health food shops.

8. **Legumes -** Look for legumes such as kidney beans, peas and soybeans. These foods contain the amino acid 'arginine' which aids in the detoxification of ammonia (by product of protein digestion).

9. **Wheatgrass -** A green drink such as wheatgrass juice or barley juice is high is chlorophyll which helps cleanse and purify the liver.

10. **Liquorice** - This herb can help to neutralise liver toxins. However, be aware that high levels of glycyrrhizic acid found in whole liquorice can be a problem for the liver. Deglycyrrhizinated or DGL is considered safer to use, so make sure you check the label.

Happy Hormone Harmony

Eat phyto-oestrogen rich foods in your daily diet if you are oestrogen deficient; alternatively include non-oestrogenic herbs such as Maca root which will help to stimulate your natural hormone production.

Eat foods rich in essential fatty acids - fish, nuts and seeds.

Include plenty of natural fibre - lentils, oats, brown rice and fruits.

Eat organic as much as possible.

Increase intake of cruciferous vegetables – cabbage, broccoli, kale, Brussel sprouts.

Drink filtered water, ironized water and calcium/magnesium rich water.

Minimise intake of white foods - sugar, flour, pasta, potatoes and rice.

Reduce intake of animal fats, milk, cheese and cream.

Limit alcohol intake.

Do not eliminate any major food groups from your diet (carbs, proteins and fats).

Chapter Four

BODY AND SOUL

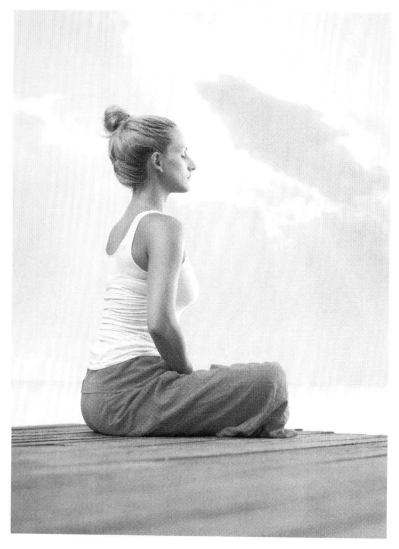

Skin Care During Menopause

As we age our skin becomes naturally drier. Our sebaceous glands produce less sebum to lubricate the skin and they are not as efficient as they were at retaining moisture. When we hit menopause the reduction of oestrogen causes a decline in elastin and collagen, which are the fibres that give support and elasticity to our skin. The decline in collagen is greatest in the years just after menopause. About 30 percent of your skin collagen is lost during the first five years after menopause and about two percent every year after that.

Genetics also play a big role in how your skin looks as you age. If your parents or older family members developed jowls, drooping eyelids and frown lines, the chances are you will too. But do bear in mind that how you take care of yourself and your skin can make a big difference in how it ages. Some of your older relatives perhaps didn't look after themselves as well as you do today, or their lifestyle was not as healthy as it could have been, especially if they were smokers. Smoking has an adverse effect on the skin, it causes biochemical changes in the body, that speeds up the ageing process. It can cause deeper wrinkles and damage the elastin in your skin.

Your Skin

The skin has many layers but it is generally divided into three main parts:

The Outer Part (Epidermis)
Has several layers and contains skin cells, pigment and proteins.

The Middle Part (Dermis)
Contains blood vessels, nerves, hair follicles and sebaceous (oil) glands. The dermis provides nutrients to the epidermis.

The Inner Layer (Subcutaneous)
Lies below the dermis and contains sweat glands, blood vessels and fat. Each layer in this section also contains connective tissue with

collagen fibres that give support and elastin that provides strength and elasticity.

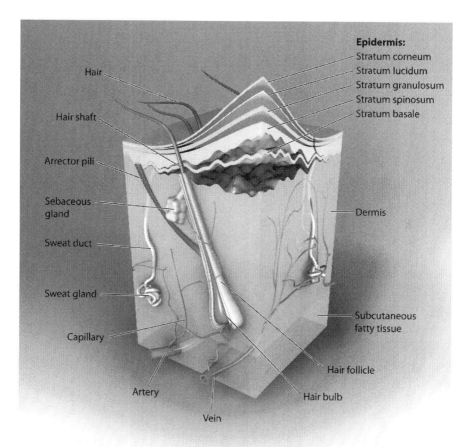

Epidermis:
Stratum corneum
Stratum lucidum
Stratum granulosum
Stratum spinosum
Stratum basale

Hair
Hair shaft
Arrector pili
Sebaceous gland
Sweat duct
Sweat gland
Capillary
Artery
Vein
Dermis
Subcutaneous fatty tissue
Hair follicle
Hair bulb

Ageing Process

Forties

During your 40's you will notice changes in your skin tone and texture. It will no longer be as tight and toned as it once was; it may look duller and pores may appear larger. You may begin to notice signs of photo-damage caused by the sun, such as age spots, discolouration and changes in skin colour. Your skin may also become dryer as hormones begin to fluctuate.

It is important to maintain a good skincare regime, and your maturing skin may need a change of products.

Fifties

Fluctuating hormones will have a more dramatic effect on your skin during your 50's. The lack of oestrogen will cause the loss of elasticity and colour and contribute towards the sagging and dryness. You will begin to notice the development of jowls and deeper lines around the eyes and mouth ,while the eyelids may have developed a crepey appearance. Brown age spots will also increase, especially in sun-exposed areas, making you more vulnerable and sensitive to the sun and it's damaging rays. Some women develop acne, particularly if they had acne during adolescence, while others may start to grow coarse facial hair.

Sixties

The change in your skin will continue through your 60's, 70's and beyond.

Once you are post-menopausal you will have a dramatic drop in oestrogen and your skin will become fine and fragile. You will need to avoid unnecessary pulling and harsh rubbing , which could lead to broken blood vessels, causing bruising and bleeding under the skin. Wrinkles and expression lines become etched into the face; your skin becomes dryer and lighter due to decreased circulation. The skin also repairs itself far more slowly than younger skin; wound healing may be up to four times slower now.

You may need to use richer creams and lotions to keep your skin hydrated.

The better you take care of your skin during your forties and fifties, the better your skin will look into its sixties and beyond.

Skin Care Regime

During the menopause transition you will probably need to adjust your skin care routine at various stages to accommodate the dryness caused by fluctuating hormones and the natural ageing process. Make sure you follow a good skin care routine to keep your skin well moisturised and minimise the effects of ageing.

Cleanse your face morning and night with your preferred cleanser; make sure it is suitable for your dryer skin. Do not use soap on your face, it is far too harsh and will strip your skin of its natural oils leaving it feeling even tighter and dryer. Face wipes have gained popularity in recent years; they are hygienic as well as being quick and easy to use. Make sure you choose ones for ageing/mature skin, preferably organic and without parabens. If your makeup is quite heavy (which hopefully it won't be) a cream/oil cleanser may be more effective. Apply to the skin and leave for a few seconds to allow it to start dissolving the makeup, wipe off using upward stokes only, never pull the skin downwards. Repeat and this time gently massage your face with the cleanser, giving yourself a mini facial at the same time and wipe off.

• Never, never, ever, ever go to bed with your make-up on - your skin will look awful the next day.
• After cleansing you may wish to tone your skin to remove any last traces of cleanser and to leave your skin feeling brighter and refreshed.
• Moisturise - You must make sure your daily moisturiser contains a SPF of at least 15 and use it every day of the year. Exposure to the sun's rays has one of the most damaging effects on the skin, and as we age we become more vulnerable, due to the lack of pigmentation in our skin.

• Use a cream at night that will keep your skin well-nourished while you sleep. If you wake in the morning and your skin feels tight, you need to change your product.

You may find that the cream you use during the day is perfectly suitable for your night time use, thus, eliminating the need to buy two separate creams.

• Anti-ageing creams - There is a lot of speculation and conflicting reports surrounding anti-ageing creams and serums and how effective they really are. They will certainly add moisture to the top layers of the skin in the epidermis and a good cream will hold moisture in and prevent that taut feeling. Some of the more advanced creams are now able to penetrate even further into the epidermis, due to the development of extremely small molecules which can be absorbed by the skin. Special active ingredients in some anti-ageing creams may also give temporary results to help minimise the appearance of wrinkles and ageing skin. Remember this is only temporary though and you will need to apply your moisturiser every day, twice a day.
• Use a gentle exfoliator once or twice a week to remove any build-up of dead skin cells, which could leave the surface of your skin looking dull.
• Use a hydrating face mask once or twice a week. This will give a boost to your moisture levels and leave your skin looking dewy and supple.
• A weekly facial and massage will help improve blood circulation and keep facial muscles toned. Treat yourself whenever you can and in between salon visits practice the home facial we have included.
• Whatever skincare regime you have for your face, apply to your neck and décolletage.

Remember it is very important to use skin care products suitable for your skin type. Most women will experience dryer skin as they age and go through the menopause. Choose something that will keep your skin hydrated and well-nourished throughout the day and night, and this doesn't mean it has to be the most expensive one or even two separate products!
Most companies are quite happy to give you samples to try, which is a good way to test the product. We are all different and what suits one may not suit the other, so try a few to see which is the most effective for you.

Keep your routine simple with:
Cleanser
Toner (Optional)
Moisturiser
Complement this with an exfoliator and a hydrating face mask.
You don't need separate eye creams; your normal moisturiser will do the job just fine. In fact if you look at the list of ingredients, they will probably be identical. The skin around the eye area is thinner so take care when applying the cream, gently pat on, and to avoid irritation don't apply too close to the eye itself.

Oestrogen Creams
May help with the appearance of ageing skin. Any cream that contains oestrogen must be prescribed by your doctor.
Certain over-the-counter creams are available that contain phyto-oestrogens (type of oestrogen contained in plants) which will help to keep your skin nourished and moisturised.
Look for the Phytomone range of products that have been specifically designed for menopausal women. They contain a carefully selected blend of some of the most beneficial botanicals and vitamins for hormonally changing skin.
If you take oestrogen pills during menopause, or any form of HT, there will be a greater production of collagen and elastin. Oestrogen will also thicken the skin. But with any hormone replacement there can be risks. Talk with your doctor about the pros and cons and weigh up the best course of action.

Vitamins For The Skin

Vitamin A
Helps in repairing skin tissue and increases cell renewal, bringing fresh new skin cells to the surface. Also known as retinol A which you are probably familiar with in skincare creams.
Include the following foods in your diet regularly to obtain vitamin A:

- Eggs
- Butter
- Lamb/beef liver
- Spinach
- Carrots
- Sweet Potatoes
- Butternut squash

Vitamin B Complex

The most important B vitamin for the skin is Biotin (B7), which forms the basis of skin, hair and nail cells. Any deficiency may result in dry, itchy skin and scalp.

Your body is capable of making biotin and it is also available in foods such as:

- Eggs
- Oatmeal
- Brown rice
- Bananas

Niacin (B3), another B vitamin helps the skin retain moisture and is found in animal sources and plants such as:

- Lean red meat
- Fish
- Pork
- Almonds
- Seeds
- Green leafy vegetable
- Carrots
- Celery

Creams containing vitamin B help to keep the skin hydrated and give a healthy glow.

Vitamin C

Helps to counter the effects of sun exposure by reducing the damage caused by free radicals, it can help the skin to appear a lot more vibrant. Include foods in your diet such as:

- Citrus fruits
- Strawberries

- Tomatoes
- Broccoli
- Cabbage
- Kiwi
- Sweet red peppers

Vitamin C in skincare products can be difficult to use due to its lack of stability. When exposed to air, vitamin C oxidises, making it not only ineffective but also potentially harmful as it may increase the formation of free radicals.

Recent research indicates that new vitamin C derivatives, consisting of multiple chemical fragments bound to a single ascorbic acid fragment, may work better. These new derivatives are more stable compared to vitamin C.

Vitamin E

Research shows that like vitamin C, vitamin E can also reduce the harmful effects of the sun on the skin. Antioxidants like vitamin E work to neutralise free radicals and stabilise cell membranes, by providing the electrons needed to complete the unstable cell. Skin cells need to be protected by antioxidants to help retain moisture in the skin and keep it looking smoother.

Food sources include:

- Almonds
- Apples
- Avocados
- Eggs
- Sunflower oil
- Sweet Potatoes
- Wheat germ oil

Vitamin E can be added to lotions, creams, and other skin care products, as well as taken orally. Free radicals are believed to play an important role in skin ageing and therefore the antioxidant activity of this vitamin is quite valuable in looking after the skin. It may help skin look younger by reducing the appearance of fine lines and wrinkles.

Minerals For The Skin

Selenium

protects from sun damage. Good dietary sources include:

- Whole grains
- Cereals
- Seafood
- Eggs
- Garlic

Copper

Together with vitamin C and zinc can help to develop elastin and keep skin supple and firm.

Good dietary sources include:

- Calf's liver
- Sesame seeds
- Cashew nuts
- Sunflower seeds
- Barley
- Navy beans

Skin creams containing copper claim they help to keep the skin firm-looking.

Zinc

Helps to keep the skin clean and can help with skin problems such as acne.

Dietary sources include:

- Oysters
- Lean meat
- Poultry

Home Facial Instructions

Try this home facial to compliment your skin care.

First, choose a good facial massage oil. Almond oil works well and is effective for mature or prematurely ageing skin.

• Open the pores to allow the benefits of a facial massage to work. If you do not own a facial steamer you can either apply wet warm towels to the face or use a bowl filled with steaming water. Place your face about 8 to 12 inches from the hot water and cover your head and the bowl with a towel to trap the heat. Steam heat the face for 5 to 10 minutes and gently pat dry.
• Apply the oil to a clean face. Use your index, middle and ring fingers to lightly stroke and massage the skin.
• Beginning at the base of the throat, use gentle upward and outward strokes, progressing with sliding movements along your jawline to the base of your ears, then use small circular motions over your cheeks and ears and around your lips.
• Now, tap your eyebrows with your middle fingers, lightly at first, and then harder. Start at the very top of the nose, and tap outwards, over the brows and then in a circular motion, around the eyes, and across the top of the cheekbones, under the eyes – until you come back up to the bridge of your nose.
• Repeat this three times, and imagine that you are 'tapping away' any stress or worry.
• Then, starting at the bridge of the nose, use the middle fingers to smooth up and outwards, in arc motions – starting small and making the arcs bigger as you move up to the top of the forehead.
• Then, open your index and middle fingers into a V-shape. Place each ear in between the V of each hand, so that the index finger is behind the ear, and the middle finger is in front, by the face.
• Press gently with both fingers, and then make small, circular motions with the middle fingers, on your temples. This is great for reducing tension headaches.
• Next, work on your nose. Begin at the hollow of each eye, and smooth down the sides of the nose with your index fingers, one on either side. Repeat this five times.
• Now starting at the top of the nose, lightly pinch down the bone, across the bridge, to the nostrils. Repeat a few times.

• Next, beginning at the centre of your forehead, use upward strokes to work your way outward with each hand, ending with circular strokes over your temples. Apply a small amount of pressure to your temples before ending your facial massage.

Other Cosmetic Procedures

Chemical Peels
This is a procedure that is used to improve and smooth the texture of the skin surface by using a chemical solution. Usually acid based, this causes the dead skin to be removed by peeling away the top layer of the epidermis. The newly generated skin is usually smoother and less wrinkled than the old skin. There are different strengths available and it is important to have a dermatologist look at your skin to evaluate your needs.

Dermabrasion
This technique uses a wire brush or a diamond wheel with rough edges to remove the upper layers of the skin. This process works by actually wounding the skin, causing it to bleed, and as the wound heals new skin grows to replace the damaged skin.
Dermabrasion is popular for the treatment of acne scars, fine lines around the mouth and age spots. This must be done by a professional person who will determine the depth of the resurfacing required, and use the appropriate pressure and coarseness of brush to obtain satisfying results.
Be aware that after this procedure the skin will be sensitive with some burning and swelling. The swelling usually goes away after about a week and the recovery time takes about 10 days.

Dermal Fillers
There are several types of dermal fillers with the most popular one being the collagen-based fillers. A dermatologist will inject the area

to be treated with the product, which will add volume and extra fullness. The most popular areas for dermal fillers are frown lines, wrinkles around the eyes and lip enhancements - be aware of the 'trout pout' and don't overdo the fillers; it could ruin your looks for life. Make sure you go to a reputable dermatologist.

Botox
Botox is a protein derived from botulism toxin, also known as botulinum. Botox works by immobilising the muscles that cause facial expressions; it is injected under the skin into the muscle to improve the look of moderate to severe frown lines or to soften wrinkles around the eyes.
It's a very popular treatment with some women having it done in their lunch hour, or even having Botox parties. Again it is important to use a professional dermatologist.

Plastic Surgery
If you want to go for a more drastic action and erase years off your face, you may want to consider plastic surgery or a surgical face-lift. Just remember there is nothing beautiful about seeing a 60 year-old woman trying to look like she is 30. If you are considering any form of plastic surgery be realistic and go for a procedure that will enhance your looks for your age and not make you look ridiculous. Keep in mind less is more, a little cosmetic surgery can be great for boosting your confidence and lifting your morale. The secret is to keep it natural looking so no one knows you've had it done.

Make-Up Box

Don't get stuck in a cosmetic time warp. If you are still wearing the same make-up as you did 20 years ago then you will look like you have come from another decade, which is not the look you want to achieve at this stage of your life.

Updating your products and colour can give you an instant glow, making you look years younger.

The best way to do this is to shcedule a cosmetic make-over. Choose a cosmetic house that you know and like. It also helps if you feel comfortable with the sales assistant and confident that she/he can give you some good advice. Although the make-over will be free of charge, they will be expecting you to buy some of their products. If you are happy with the advice they have given and pleased with the look they have created for you, then consider it a good investment. But do not feel obliged to buy anything at all if you are not happy with the end result. Stand your ground, be confident and explain why you are not happy. Do not be rail-roaded into buying anything. If you do, you will get home, the products will stay in the drawer and you will feel frustrated with yourself for wasting so much money. Yes, you want their advice, but you must also feel comfortable with your new look. If they haven't managed to do this then they have failed to do their job properly.

Things You Will Need In Your New Make-Up Bag

Skin Illuminator

Can make a real difference to the look of your skin. These products contain microscopic particles that act like tiny mirrors to reflect light onto your skin, resulting in a bright, radiant complexion. They are available in creams, liquids and powders. To emphasise the glow choose products tinted light peach or warm beige tones. Ask the make-up consultant which tones best suit your skin.

Concealers

Will cover any discolouration around the eye area caused by thinning skin and menopausal sleepless nights and cover any small broken veins, brown spots or blemishes that may be starting to appear. Choose a good concealer that blends well with your natural skin tone. Avoid ultra-light colours and ensure it doesn't emphasise any fine lines around the eye area. You may need to experiment with a few before you find the right one and a texture you like, but the effort will be worth it and the end result could take years off you. Apply concealer after foundation; you might be surprised at how little you need. Waterproof concealers are available if you're suffering from hot flushes.

Tinted Moisturisers

These products combine the benefits of skin care and a light foundation for a natural luminous complexion. They will add a slight tint to enhance your natural skin tone, giving you a healthy glow with an 'un-made up' look and the added benefit of keeping your skin moisturised. Make sure you use one that has an SPF to protect your skin from sun damage.

Bronzers

Can add a glorious glow to your skin and are a perfect choice for mid-life, since this is when we tend to lose colour from our faces which can add years to our appearance. Choose a bronzer no more than two shades darker than your natural skin tone. If you have fair skin go for one with yellow/peach undertones and dark skins should go for warm reds/brown tones. Ask for advice if you are unsure which one to go for. Never apply bronzer all over your face, dust it over the high points where the sun would naturally catch your skin, such as top of cheek bones, and down the centre of the nose. Blend upwards towards your temples and sweep across your forehead with a very light dusting into the hairline, blending it in well.

Foundations

Will give you more coverage and hide minor imperfections. Choose a moisturising foundation that has an SPF and one that won't dry out your skin. A soft dewy complexion will be far more flattering than a heavily made up face. Choose a colour that matches your complexion, or a very subtle shade darker if you feel you need a little more colour. Do not be tempted to go for much darker shades to add colour to your face, this will look un-naturally obvious and will draw attention for the wrong reasons.

Make sure you blend the foundation well around the jaw line and neck area and look for a sweat proof foundation if you're suffering from hot flushes.

Powders
Can be unforgiving and accentuate wrinkles and facial hair. If you like the matte look powders offer, choose a mineral powder in a translucent shade. This will give the most natural look and the minerals will help absorb any excess oil or moisture.

Eye shadows
A professional make-up consultant should be able to give you advice on colours, textures and how to apply them to achieve the most effective results. However, make sure you stay away from creamy frosted or shimmery eye shadows; they will settle in the creases of your eyelid and accentuate any crepey skin. Avoid bright colours and choose warm earthy tones with maybe two or three complimentary colours in the pallet. Use the lighter shade on the inner half of the eyelid and blend the darker shade on the outer half, taking it slightly underneath the outer corner of the eye to give a soft smoky look and the appearance of the eye being larger.

Eyeliners
Can give more definition to the eyes, but keep it soft looking with a 'smudge' effect otherwise it may look too severe. Black can be harsh, choose softer shades such as browns, greens, blues or grey.

Mascara
Finish your eye make-up off with mascara. Again black can be harsh, brown/black or brown will be far more complimentary. Choose a volumising mascara, and apply two coats making sure you cover lashes in the outer corner of your eyes to make them look wider. This can be a bit tricky, so try using just the tip of the mascara wand to separate and coat these lashes. If you're suffering from hot flushes, avoid the 'panda' look by choosing waterproof mascara.

Tip: you may find your eyelashes become quite sparse during the menopause; if you feel you need a little more natural volume but don't wont to wear false eyelashes, look out for the individual lashes that can be applied to the outer corners of the eyes or in places where you need that extra fullness. They can be fiddly to apply to begin with and you may need to practice a little, or if you find it too time consuming, most beauty salons offer this treatment.

Eyebrow Pencils

Avoid harsh eyebrow pencils that give that 'drawn on' effect and can make you look like some sort of cartoon character. Use powders or a soft pencil and very lightly apply in the opposite direction of the hair growth, then brush eyebrows into place with an eyebrow brush, blending in the pencil.

Blushers

Like bronzers will help to contour your face and add colour. Choose soft shades of peaches and coral browns. Avoid bright colours and anything with sparkles.
Apply to cheekbone area and sweep up towards the temples, finishing with a very fine dusting along the hairline to add warmth.

Lips

Can look fuller by using a lip pencil but make sure it is the same colour as your lipstick. Heavy outlined lips are not an attractive look. Go for soft warm shades of coral and reds. Dark colours can accentuate any problems and make you look harsh, also avoid bright colours and frosted lipsticks.
Look after your lips by using a gentle lip scrub which will remove any dry skin and help improve the circulation, bringing more blood to your lips and giving a fuller 'plumper' look. Use a lip balm when not wearing a lipstick to keep your lips soft and smooth.

Hair Care

During menopause you may find that your hair becomes thinner and may even fall out, not only on your head but legs, arms and pubic hair may also be affected.
The two main hormones involved in hair growth are oestrogen and testosterone. Oestrogen helps hair grow faster and stay in the head longer; testosterone can shrink hair follicles causing hair loss.
The low levels of oestrogen during menopause mean less oil is produced in the scalp and other areas. Nearly every hair follicle is

attached to a sebaceous gland and without oil some hair follicles can cease to function, hair is lost and not replaced.

In some women the testosterone imbalance can cause more hair to grow, but not necessarily in the places we want it, such as on the face and chest. It will also be coarser than your other hair.

There are some over-the-counter products you can buy to help with thinning hair such as Regaine. The active ingredient in this is minoxidil, which helps to enlarge and lengthen hair follicles, extending the growth phase. It doesn't cure hair loss but it can slow down the process. Ketoconozole is another active ingredient which helps reduce the amount of androgen hormones (testosterone), and stops the hair follicles from shrinking. It also helps you retain your existing hair for longer. When buying over-the-counter products for hair loss, look out for these two ingredients, because without them they will have no effect. Some companies will add ingredients that cause a tingling sensation on the scalp to make the product feel as if it is working, but this is no more than a sensation. Talk to your dermatologist for more advice on these hair treatments.

Wigs and Hair Pieces
Can look very natural and come in a wide range of styles and colours. If your hair loss is making you unhappy, this could be just what you need to improve your confidence and self-image.

Grey Hair
Hair goes grey when the pigment cells containing melanin, which rest at the base of each hair follicle, start to die off and the pigment in each follicle begins to diminish.

Grey hair can look very elegant, though it will be coarser in texture and may need more looking after. If the silver fox look suits you, stay with it, get a good haircut and use lots of moisturising products. If you're not comfortable with your grey hair and feel it is ageing you too much too soon, then there is a plethora of products out there to choose from, or get more advice from you hairdresser.

Hair Care Recipes

Scalp Massage Oil

2 tsps. (10ml) base oil – coconut is a good choice
3 drops sandalwood oil
3 drops rosemary or jasmine oil

Gently heat base oil in a small cup or bowl in microwave or double saucepan, mix in essential oils.

Pour a little oil into your palm, rub it into the crown of your head, apply a little more oil, rake your fingers down from the crown of your head to your ears and then from the crown of your head to the nape of your neck.

Now massage your scalp by using small firm circular movements with your finger-tips and cover the entire scalp. Make sure your movements are firm enough to stimulate the scalp.

Wrap your hair in cling film and then cover your head with a hot towel and relax for 20 minutes before shampooing – or if possible, leave on overnight, cover your pillow with a towel and wear a soft shower cap.

Cream Hair Bath

½ cup (125ml) coconut oil
2 Tbsp. coconut cream
5 drops eucalyptus oil
5 drops rose oil
5 drops rosemary oil

Heat coconut oil until warm, remove from heat and add coconut cream, stir well and add essential oils.
Massage into the scalp and hair and wrap a hot towel around your head. Leave to absorb for 30 minutes.
Shampoo well, rinse and condition as usual.

Wild Lime Hair Rinse

Juice of 2 limes
1 cup (250ml) distilled water
Squeeze lime juice from the limes and add to water, stir well and use
as a weekly rinse after shampooing

Apply conditioner as usual.

Fragrant Hair Serum

5 drops essential oil of choice
3 drops coconut or jojoba oil

Mix together and place in palm of hand, rub palms together and
gently scrunch into damp hair - make sure you distribute oils evenly,
paying special attention to ends of the hair. Dry as normal.

Top Foods For Healthy Hair

To keep your hair looking its very best, eating a well-balanced diet is
crucial. Crash diets or fad diets that have you eliminate certain food
groups and nutrients can lead to dull dry hair and even hair loss.

Chicken: Excellent source of protein to strengthen hair strands, and
B6 which contributes to cell renewal and red blood cell health to
carry oxygen to the scalp.

Fish: Is a good source of protein, which the hair is primarily made
up of. Omega 3 in salmon will help nourish the scalp, and B12 found
in trout will promote red blood cell functions and help the hair form
protein tissue.

Lentils: Will also help to keep red blood cells healthy, so they can
carry oxygen to the scalp and skin.

Walnuts: Excellent source of fatty acids (omega 3). Walnuts help
maintain hair texture and prevent dry brittle hair.

Pumpkin Seeds: Contain magnesium which helps prevent hair loss. Our body cannot make magnesium so we must get it from our diet.

Beef: Good source of zinc which we need for hair growth and maintaining colour. A deficiency can lead to hair loss and premature ageing.

Eggs: Egg yolks are rich in biotin, a B vitamin which metabolises fatty acids to fuel growth and repair of hair follicles. But the eggs must be cooked in order for the body to absorb the biotin.

Carrots: Are very high in beta-carotene, which the body converts into vitamin A. Carrots are a great food for your hair. Vitamin A promotes sebum production so the hair is moisturised with the right amount of natural oils.

Sunflower Seeds: High in vitamin E, a nutrient that promotes blood flow to the scalp, which aids hair growth.

Water: Makes up a quarter of the weight of a strand of hair. When hair has the proper amount of water it will respond by being supple and shiny.

Facial Hair

Unwanted facial hair is caused by the imbalance of oestrogen and testosterone and can sprout up not only on the face but also the neck, chest and other odd places.

If it's not too severe, using your tweezers is a quick and effective way to get rid of it. Pull in the direction of the hair growth to make sure it comes out at the root, ensuring re-growth is slow. Do not shave facial hair.

Hair Bleach – Can be effective if you have fine facial hair.

Waxing – Is an alternative to using your tweezers and may be quicker if you have more than the odd hair to pull out; like tweezing, waxing pulls your hair out from the root giving a slower re-growth time.

Electrolysis – Offers a permanent way to remove unwanted hair. A small, fine needle is inserted into the hair follicle and a strong electrical current is applied. This kills the root of the hair and destroys the hair follicle so it can no longer grow anymore hair.

Pubic Hair

Can become thin or patchy for much the same reasons as hair loss on your head. Most women are quite happy to live with it, while others wax to minimise the effect and some have laser treatment or electrolysis to permanently remove what's left. It's a personal choice so go with whatever makes you feel happy.

Perfect Pampering

Let's not forget it's not just the skin of our face that is ageing. The rest of our body is too and it needs just as much looking after and pampering.

Bathing

Bathing can be a wonderful experience, especially when combined with oils, candles, soft music and incense. It can help ease away the aches and pains of the day and dissolve menopausal symptoms.

It can be your personal spiritual retreat, a place to contemplate in solitude.

You can create a spa inspired bathroom with just a few simple changes. Natural materials work well to create a spa atmosphere. Choose things such as bamboo floor mats and other warm textured accessories like rattan chairs and baskets to hold rolled hand towels, wash cloths and bath items. Cane or wicker shelving units are ideal for storing bulky towels. Use white towels and bath robes for a crisp, clean feel.

Bring a touch of nature into your spa bathroom with flowers and plants. Just one giant fern in the corner by the bath means you can fantasise that your shower is really an exotic outdoor waterfall. Hanging baskets can also be extremely effective in creating that outdoor shower illusion. Make sure you choose something suitable for the humid conditions of the bathroom. Don't use plants with soft or velvety leaves, the steam and moisture will cause the plant to die. The following plants usually do well in bathrooms:

Philodendron: These cascading plants are easy to grow and are ideal for hanging baskets or pots.
Ficus: This includes the ficus benjamina, better known as the weeping fig, which does well in pots.
Bamboo: It is not only a plant associated with good luck, but also does well in humid places.

Others to try include spider plant, ferns, asparagus fern (this plant is not a fern, but a member of the lily family), begonia, grape ivy, orchid and gardenia.

Keep your bathroom sparking clean and have plenty of spa products, ingredients and accessories to play with. Bath salts and essential oils are the staples, while more exotic additions may be picked up on your travels.

Try to find time once or twice a week to indulge in this unhurried luxury. Remove any distractions - partner, kids, pets - take the phone off the hook and disappear into your sanctuary.

Surround yourself with candles and dim the lights. If you are taking your bath in the evening burn a relaxing oil such as sandalwood to help easy away the stresses of the day and play soft soothing music for the soul. Have a glass of water with a slice of lemon – or if it's been a particularly hard day, a glass of wine. Have your big fluffy towels close by and your robe ready to slip into.

If you are taking your bath in the morning, use energising ingredients to begin your day with vibrancy. While winter baths taken in the early afternoon as the rain is pouring down makes for a most nurturing journey, sip hot tea and have your luscious warm towels to hand.

Prepare your bath, making sure it's not too hot. Add a few drops of essential oil of your choice to the water and inhale the vapours. Essential oils will help nourish the skin and give a sense of well-being. Alternatively, you may like to use bath milk, herbs, salts or your own personal favourite.

Before you step into your bath spend a few moments just breathing. Breathe deeply and exhale the tensions that have built up within you. Look at the flame of your candle and focus your thoughts, and then allow them to drift away. Now step into your bath, be aware of your body slipping gently into the water, sense how it feels as it caresses your skin, the soft-scented water enveloping your body and gently melting away the aches and pains of the day; breathe in the scent of the oils and allow them to relax your mind.

Enjoy the ambiance of this sanctuary- like space you have created. Nothing else matters right now, just you, in your space, in your time, in your world. Relax and allow everything to drift out of your mind.

Bath Recipes

Flower petal Bath
Simple and exotic – just add a few drops of your favourite essential oils along with some fresh flower petals – looks amazing and smells divine. Try mixing the following blends together and adding to your bath

Tropical Rain:
1 Tbsp. (20ml) coconut oil/jojoba oil or similar
12 drops ylang ylang essential oil
12 drops jasmine essential oil

12 drops clove essential oil

Morning Mist :
1 Tbsp. (20ml) coconut oil/ jojoba oil or similar
12 drops ginger essence
12 drops ylang ylang essential oil
12 drops jasmine essential oil

Warmest Wishes:
1 Tbsp. (20ml) coconut oil/jojoba or similar
12 drops nutmeg essential oil
12 drops cinnamon essential oil
12 drops clove essential oil

Herb Bath Bags

If you don't like the idea of sharing your bath water with herbs, spices and flowers but still want to enjoy their delicious smells and moisturising benefits, try using a bath bag. These are normally filled with a selection of scented herbs and dried flowers and maybe oatmeal or bath salts. You can buy these little muslin bags ready-made or they are simple enough to make. All you need is a square of muslin or any other light fabric, ribbon and one cup of your pot-pourri mix. Place the pot-pourri mix in the middle of the square cloth, tie together with ribbon or band, and place in your bath under the running water - simple and effective.

Recipe Ideas

9" x 9" square muslin or similar
Ribbon
2 Tbsp. lavender buds
2 Tbsp. chamomile flowers
2 Tbsp. rose petals
1 Tbsp. oatmeal
5 drops essential oil

Mix together and make into bag, tie with ribbon - long enough to hang from hot water tap so water can flow through.

There are many variations you can try. Have fun experimenting , add your favourite oils to the mix to create the mood you desire. Use a variety of herbs, spices, fruits and flowers. Use oatmeal as a softener, Dead Sea salts for their rich mineral properties, or even add dried milk powder for a silky smooth bath.

Milk Baths
Milk baths were made legendary by Cleopatra. The milk and its derivatives contain lactic acid which help to dissolve the proteins which hold dead skin cells together, making it a great exfoliator.

Basic Milk and Honey Bath Recipe
½ cup liquid honey
2 cups powdered milk
Lavender buds or rose buds for colour and fragrance
6-10 drops essential oil

Combine these ingredients together, add to bath water or transfer into a decorative bottle and keep in your bathroom until ready to use.

Simple Milk Bath Recipe
1 cup powdered milk
2-3 drops favourite essential oil
Mix together and add to bath water

If you find your skin is too oily after a milk bath, try using a low fat version or powdered soymilk.

Soymilk and Mandarin Bath
This bath may help alleviate some of your menopausal symptoms. It is perfect if you feel a little stressed or off- centre. It will help balance body temperature and stimulate, soften and hydrate the skin. Oatmeal is a good skin softener, mandarin is an emotionally-balancing and serene oil and the milk is hydrating and exfoliating.

1 cup (125g) hydrated soymilk
1 Tbsp. oatmeal
1 Tbsp. mandarin or orange citrus peel

¼ cup sea salt
10 drops mandarin essential oil

Blend oatmeal, citrus peel and sea salt together in food processor until it has consistency of fine powder. Then mix with the hydrated soymilk. Prepare warm bath and dissolve the ingredients into the water, adding the essential oil drops last, alternatively add the essential oil to the sea salt before mixing.

Rejuvenating Himalayan Bath Ritual

2 Tbsp. (40ml) Tibetan/Himalayan salts (substitute with Dead Sea salts if unavailable)
1 Tbsp. (20ml) plain salt
1 cup (250ml) dried herbs such as nettle, ginger, neem and coriander
4 drops juniper essential oil
4 drops mandarin essential oil
4 drops grapefruit essential oil

Mix together and add to warm bath . Relax and enjoy. Have a small decorative pouring jug or jar to pour bath water gently over yourself.

Bath Salts

We all know that our bodies are made up mostly of water, as well as salt and various other minerals and proteins.
When salt is in a solution such as water, it is able to penetrate our cellular walls and help flush out toxins from the body and improve our circulation. Sea salts and Epsom salts are the best choice to use for bathing.

As well as being a therapeutic aid in the relief of sore muscles and aching joints, bath salts cleanse the skin and help remove excess oil and toxins, and when bath salts are mixed with essential oils they can help promote even greater relaxation. They are also a favourite choice for exfoliators and scrubs.

So to enhance your bathing experience, add some bath salts to the water. Try the Phytomone range of hormone balancing bath crystals and let the aches and pains of the day disappear and your stress slip away as you relax in the fragrant warm water.

No more wrinkling skin
The outer layer of our skin is capable of absorbing water and when we lie in the bath it soaks up the water and starts to swell. As the skin is thickest on the hands and feet, it absorbs the most water, and eventually the skin will start to buckle and fold into wrinkles.
Bath salts change the osmotic balance of the water, so less water is absorbed by the skin via osmosis.
This reduces the 'wrinkling' effect we get on the skin, especially on our fingers when we have been in the bath a little too long.

Dry Body Brushing

Daily body brushing is an invigorating experience. It will wake your skin up and leave you feeling very refreshed.
As most of us know by now, our skin is the largest organ we have and it is responsible for a quarter of the body's detoxification each day.
Dry brushing the skin helps to improve the circulation and remove dead skin cells, as well as:

Cleanses the lymphatic system.
Strengthens the immune system.
Stimulates the hormones and oil- producing glands.
Tightens skin, preventing premature ageing.
Tones muscles.

Choose a soft natural fibre brush (synthetic fibres are too sharp and may damage your skin) Make sure it has a long handle so you can reach all parts of your body. You can change to a coarser brush once your skin becomes used to it. Both your skin and the brush must be dry.

Start at your feet and brush upwards towards your heart, using long sweeping strokes Stroking away from your heart puts pressure on the valves within the veins and lymph vessels and can cause ruptured vessels and varicose veins.

Work your way up your body, brushing every part of your skin. Use light pressure in areas where your skin is thin, and harder pressure in areas like the soles of your feet. Avoid sensitive areas and anywhere the skin is broken, such as cuts, wounds or infections. Try to brush your skin for about 10 minutes each day to improve circulation and slough off dead skin cells. Finish with a shower or bath to remove impurities and massage an oil or cream into your skin to keep it nourished.

Keep your body brush clean by washing it once a week with a mild soap. Dry in a sunny spot to prevent mildew.

Body Scrubs

Are a great way to keep your skin healthy and beautiful. A good quality scrub will cleanse and exfoliate the skin, sloughing off dead skin cells and moisturise at the same time.
By massaging the body scrub into your skin you will be improving the blood circulation, leaving your skin looking radiant and glowing.

Use a body scrub once or twice a week, if you use it more often, the frequent scrubbing may damage the young skin cells as most dead skin has already been removed.
Body scrubs at a spa are always a good treatment to have as the therapist will work longer massaging it in and will also be able to reach difficult areas.
But in between spa treatments why not have a go at making your own body scrub – The basic ingredients for any body scrub will be:

1. **An exfoliant** – such as salt, sugar, rice, coffee grounds, apricot kernels etc. to rub away the dead skin cells on the surface, leaving smoother, softer skin.

2. Oil - This helps hold the mixture together so you can apply it to your skin. It also helps keep the skin soft and hydrated. Choose a good- quality oil such as jojoba, grape seed, sweet almond or even olive oil. I would not recommend mineral oil because this will not penetrate into the skin like other oils will. Mineral oil is pore clogging and once it evaporates, your skin may be left looking dryer than before you used it.

3. Fragrance - Should come from high quality essential oils which are beneficial to the skin and have a lasting aroma.

The budget variety of body scrubs available probably use synthetic fragrances and lower quality oils. If you are going to go to the trouble of using a body scrub use good quality ingredients that will have a beneficial effect on the body.

Salt scrubs and sugar scrubs are by far the most popular on the market.

Salt tends to offer more therapeutic benefits, while removing impurities and toxins as it polishes your skin. The mineralising properties of salt are also extremely beneficial, though they do tend to be slightly more abrasive than sugar scrubs.

Sugar scrubs are a little gentler and may be better if you have sensitive skin. They tend to be less drying and the granules dissolve more readily, making them less abrasive, but they do not contain the mineralising benefits of salt scrubs.

Coffee scrubs have been popular in Asia for many years and can normally be found on spa menus, but they are still not that easy to come by in the high street. The coffee bean actually contains magnesium and vitamin E. which acts as an anti-oxidant and has bacterial, exfoliating and stimulating properties.

Body Scrub Recipes

Basic Scrub

½ cup (125ml) coarse brown sugar
1 cup (250ml) grape seed oil
4 Tbsp. (80ml) grated lemon peel

Mix all ingredients together, gently rub on body in circular motion.
Pay attention to rough areas like elbows and knees, rinse with water.

Coconut and Ginger Shred

½ cup (125ml) base oil (such as almond, grape seed, olive oil)
½ (125ml) cup desiccated coconut flakes
1 Tbsp. (20ml) fresh ginger finely grated

Grind coconut flakes in grinder; mix all ingredients together in a
bowl. Rub all over body massaging vigorously to stimulate
circulation. Step into the shower, allowing the water to further
hydrate the skin then rinse off well.

Lemon Salt Glow

½ cup (125ml)sea salt
½ cup (125ml) sweet almond oil
1 Tbsp. (20ml) finely grated lemon zest
10 drops ginger essential oil

Add oil slowly to the salt. The mixture should not be too oily, but
not too dry either. Adapt amount to get required consistency, stir in
essential oil and then add lemon zest. Store in an air-tight container
in a cool dry place until ready to use.

Coffee Scrub

2 cups (500ml) coarse ground coffee
½ cup (125ml) Natural brown sugar

¼ cup (60ml) olive oil
5 drops ylang ylang essential oil (or oil of choice)

Combine all ingredients, rub mixture into skin in large circular movements, paying attention to problem areas, shower and follow with body lotion.

Adding bentonite or kaolin clay (cosmetic grade) and seaweed will help detoxify and purify the skin. Honey will add moisture and baking soda will add vibrant sparkle.

If you are feeling creative or making the body scrubs as a gift for someone, adding herbs and flowers will make it look more attractive as well as adding additional exfoliation.

Body Moisturisers

A good moisturiser is one of your skin's best friends. Water constantly evaporates through our skin into the air at the rate of about one pint per day and the more water our skin loses the drier it gets.

All body lotions, creams, butters and oils - whether rich and heavy or light and silky - will form a film on your skin that adds a barrier, helping to seal in moisture for longer and prevent evaporation. They will also give your skin a subtle glow and a scent that lingers for hours.

An effective moisturiser should contain an oil or an oil- like substance that spreads smoothly to create an even layer over the skin surface.

The main types of oils used in skin care creams and lotions are vegetable oils such as almond, avocado, coconut, olive and palm to name just a few. Many vegetable oils are readily absorbed by the top layers of the skin.

Happy Feet

Of all our body parts, our feet tend to suffer most. We stuff them into shoes and pay little respect to the fact that they carry our whole body weight. One quarter of all our body's bones (26) are in our feet and they deserve just as much attention as any other part of our body. There is nothing worse than sore feet, but if we don't look after them what can we expect?

After a challenging day, pamper your feet with this Foot Spa Ritual:

Foot Spa Ritual

Choose a large, visually-pleasing earthenware bowl for bathing your feet; this will enhance your foot spa experience.
In the bottom of the bowl put a collection of small river stones (available from crafts stores or garden centers) or medium- sized marbles.
Fill the bowl with warm water and add 3 drops of thyme essential oil, 3 drops vetiver oil and 3 drops sage oil.
Sprinkle fresh flower petals on the top.

Lower feet one by one into the bowl and soak for 15-20 minutes. During this time gently roll your feet back and forth over the stones/marbles, occasionally grasp and release the stones/marbles with your toes. This action stretches and releases the feet.

After soaking, scrub each foot gently with a pumice stone to remove hard skin, concentrating on the heels and ball of the feet. Alternatively, you may like to use a foot scrub to exfoliate and remove hard skin. There are many to choose from on the high street, or make a simple one yourself using a handful of coarse sea salt mixed with a vegetable oil to make a paste and add five drops of either peppermint oil, sage or cypress oil. Scrub each foot with the mixture and return to the bowl.

For a refreshing end to your foot spa, have a jug of cold water at hand. Take your feet out of the bowl one at a time and pour the cold water over to rinse and refresh.
Wrap your feet in a warm towel and pat dry.

Now you can massage your feet with a cream, lotion or oil to relax the muscles, stimulate circulation and oxygenate the blood.

This is also a good time to trim your toe nails, as they will be soft after your foot spa. Trim them straight across, not too short and don't round off at the outside corners too much, as it could result in an in-growing toe nail.
Push cuticles back gently with an orange stick and either buff or add your nail polish.

Finally put on a pair of cotton socks to protect your pampered feet.

Hands

Many of us take great care of our faces, but forget all about our ageing hands. Next to our faces, our hands are probably the most visible part of our body.
The skin on the back of our hands is very thin and delicate, there is almost no fat or collagen under it at all, and what there is decreases as we grow older. The skin becomes dry and loose and you may notice age spots starting to develop.
Our hands need extra care otherwise they will begin to show the signs of age well before our faces do.

Test your age:
Try this experiment to see what your skin's biological age is and to test the elasticity or stretch ability of your skin.
Pinch the skin on the back of your hand and then release it after a few seconds.
Under 30 and the skin should return quickly to its original contour.
Between 30- 50 you will probably notice the skin stand up for a second or two before recovering.
50 and beyond the skin may stand up for a number of seconds.

Looking after your hands should be part of your daily skincare regime; if it isn't, start now.

Begin cultivating graceful, well-cared for hands by dedicating a few minutes each day to cleansing, moisturising and self-massaging. Choose creams that have lightening agents in them to reduce the effect of any age spots.
Reflex points exist in the hand area, and they respond well to regular massage, which will keep them nourished and toned. Hand massage also increases circulation, keeps joints flexible and skin looking soft and smooth. Don't forget to do the hand exercises.

Hand Care Ritual

Cleanse
Pour a few drops of lemongrass essential oil into warm water and relax your hands for a few minutes. The lemongrass will help soothe and heal the hands as well as act as a natural antiseptic.

Hand scrub
To gently get rid of dead skin cells while nourishing your skin use a mild exfoliator – try mixing together:

2 Tbsp. (40ml) dried coconut or freshly grated coconut
2 Tbsp. (40ml) coconut cream (or your regular hand cream)

Mix together and use small circular movements on back of hands.

Rosewater Hand Mask
Use this softening hand wrap to leave hands smooth, hydrated and nourished.

2 Tbsp. (40ml) rosewater
3 Tbsp. (60ml) oatmeal
2 Tbsp. (40ml) almond oil

Mix all ingredients together and heat in a double saucepan until warm.
Apply the warm mask to the back of the hands (not the palm), wrap in cling film or warm towels and leave for 10 minutes - rinse off and pat dry.

Simple Hand Massage

Try this self-massage to rebalance energy levels and promote relaxation. Try the recipe below or even blend one of your own. Alternatively, use a rich hand cream.

4 Tbsp. wheat germ oil
5 drops thyme essential oil
5 drops eucalyptus essential oil
5 drops lime essential oil

Mix well together.

• Apply a small amount of the oil/cream to the back of you left hand, using smooth strokes from your fingertips up to your wrist.

• Turn your left hand over, cupping it with your right hand, and with your thumb use small circular movements to massage the palm of your left hand. Add more oil or cream as you need it. Briefly press the centre of your palm to promote relaxation.

• Turn your left hand over , and starting at your little finger, use your thumb to apply small circular massage movements to each knuckle, working down each finger. When you get to the fingertip briefly squeeze to stimulate the brain and promote clear thinking.

• Repeat this procedure on your right hand.

• Finish by flexing your fingers and shaking your hands.

• Apply a rich hand cream last thing at night and then slip on a pair of cotton gloves. Wear them as you sleep to seal in moisture and keep your hand luxuriously soft and smooth.

Essential Oils

Essential oils are a very pleasant way to lift your moods and help you to relax at the same time.

Most oils have several different properties and each person may respond slightly differently. Try experimenting with different oils to find which suit you best.

Several essential oils contain a hormone-like substance related to oestrogen and may be helpful during menopause. These include: Clary sage, anise, fennel, cypress, coriander, geranium, lavender, neroli, rose and sage.

Other useful essential oils:

Hot Flushes
Peppermint, lemon, clary sage, cypress oil.

Moods
Chamomile, jasmine, neroli, frankincense, basil, sweet marjoram.

Fatigue
Basil, clary sage, ginger.

Relaxing
Lavender, sweet marjoram.

Uplifting
Ylang ylang, rosemary, grapefruit, lemongrass, ginger.

Blending

The general rule of thumb for blending essential oils is to use six drops of essential oil to every two tsps. (10ml) of carrier oil. Remember essential oils are highly concentrated and can be toxic if used incorrectly. A little oil will go a long way.

You can have lots of fun experimenting and blending oils together. Each oil has its own individual character and as you become more familiar with the different oils you will learn and understand which oils blend well with each other. A good blend will have a top note, a middle note and a base note, making it balanced and well-rounded.

Top Notes
Are the most volatile. They are the first that we smell, but tend to dissipate quickly. They tend to be light and fresh such as lemon, bergamot and eucalyptus.

Middle Notes
Represent the heart of the fragrance. You will pick up the smell of a middle note after the top notes and it will linger a while longer. Middle notes are oils such as neroli, lavender, rosemary, geranium and rosewood.

Base Notes
These are rich and heavy and last a long time. In perfumery, base notes are known as fixatives, as they literally fix a perfume and hold it together, helping to prevent the lighter notes from dispersing too quickly. Essential oils for base notes may include patchouli, myrrh, sandalwood, and frankincense.

.

Essential Oil Recipes

Start by trying some of the blends included here, or choose just three or four oils of your preference to begin so you don't get too overwhelmed.

An egg cup is ideal for blending - experiment and have fun.

Blend One
4 tsps. (20ml) base oil
4 drops frankincense
4 drops myrrh
4 drops sandalwood

Blend Two
4 tsps. (20ml) base oil
5 drops neroli
5 drops lavender
2 drops geranium

Blend Three
4 tsps. (20ml) base oil
4 drops sandalwood
4 drops jasmine
4 drops bergamot

Blend Four
4 tsps. (20ml) base oil
5 drops rose absolute
4 drops sandalwood
3 drops patchouli

Think of rose and lavender when you want to create an ambiance of calm; try citrus fruits with a dash of black pepper for uplifting and enlivening; for relaxing go for an earthy blend such as sandalwood and vetiver, and for motivation choose oils like rosemary and peppermint.

There are many essential oils to choose from, and the beauty of blending various oils is that it's really up to you. Follow your nose and don't be afraid to be adventurous. Be creative in your mixing and have fun.

Body Oils
These can be used on a daily basis and are good to use after a shower or bath to help seal in moisture.
Try the body oil from the Phytomone range, this light fragrant oil is perfect for hormonally changing skin.

Body Mists
Are light and refreshing and can cool you off during a hot flush or have a warming effect during the winter, depending on the oils you use.
Remember not to use plastic bottles as the essential oils can chemically react with the plastic. You will need to shake the bottle well every time before use as oils don't dissolve in water, and you might like to add vodka or pure alcohol to the spray to assist with this. The alcohol is entirely optional and will act as a preservative. Pour your chosen blend below into a clean bottle with a spray nozzle, secure lid and shake well.

Body Mist
8fl.oz. distilled water
2 Tbsp. (30ml) vodka (optional)
6 drops sandalwood oil
6 drops rose oil
4 drops vanilla oil
3 drops jasmine oil

Hot Flush Mist
4fl.oz. distilled water
24 drops clary sage oil
48 drops peppermint Oil
24 drops geranium oil
24 drops lemon oil
Try massaging peppermint oil into soles of feet or back of neck for a cooling effect.

Room Sprays

Room sprays are an alternative way to fragrance you home and can be made up using water and essential oils.

Base Ingredients

50ml distilled water
50ml vodka or ethanol (rubbing alcohol)
20 drops essential oils of choice

Mood-Enhancing Room Spray

50ml distilled water
50ml vodka or ethanol (rubbing alcohol)
5 drops sandalwood
5 drops frankincense
5 drops chamomile
5 drops cedar wood

You might like to try rosewood and bergamot for living areas; for the bathroom try cedar wood and pine, and for the bedroom try rose, patchouli, mandarin and sandalwood.

Experiment with different oils to get the blend you prefer.

Sleep Sprays

Disturbed sleep during the menopause can leave you feeling exhausted. Try these natural sleep inducers instead of taking sleep medications.

Night Time Bliss

10ml (2tsps) distilled water
4 drops lavender
3 drops jasmine
1 drop ylang ylang

Put into spray bottle, shake well and spritz pillow. Alternatively, just sprinkle one or two drops of lavender oil onto your pillow.

Essential Oils For Your Home

Pomanders
Hang or place small porous corked bottles in your wardrobe, fill with fragrance of your choice. The essential oil is absorbed by the clay and released slowly.

Shoe Rack
Freshen up your cupboard with lemongrass.
Deodorise shoes with two drops of pine or parsley oil.

Wood Fires
Sprinkle drops of cypress, cedar wood, pine or sandalwood over the logs to be used about an hour before lighting the fire and then burn to release to aroma.

Vacuum Cleaners
Put 4- 6 drops of oil onto a cotton wool ball and place in dust bag or cylinder. This freshens and perfumes the room while you are cleaning and keeps the vacuum smelling pleasant.

Scented Candles
Are always a popular choice to scent a room and add ambiance. Most candles are already infused with a fragrance, but for a stronger smell, try adding a few drops of oil to the candle wick before lighting.

Scented Liners
Place paper tissues scented with essential oils in linen cupboards between sheets, pillow cases and towels to gently perfume them. Also use in bedroom draws.
Try a mixture of lavender, ylang ylang and bergamot.

Headaches
Make a cold compress using lavender and peppermint and apply to head.

Toothache
Put a drop of clove oil on a cotton wool bud and apply to affected area. Clove is an analgesic, helping to relieve pain.

Burns
Cool skin by using ice cold water for at least five minutes; apply neat lavender oil to affected area. Lavender will reduce pain and provide rapid healing.

Fragrance Oils
These are not the same as essential oils - so don't be fooled. Fragrance oils are artificially created fragrances and contain artificial substances, or they are essential oils that have been diluted with carrier oils.
They do not offer the calibre or therapeutic benefits that essential oils do.

FEED YOUR SOUL

Meditation

Meditation is the way to bring us back to ourselves, so we can really experience and taste our full being. In the stillness and silence of meditation, we can return to that deep inner nature that we have so long ago lost sight of amid the busyness and distraction of our minds.

Meditation is about appreciating and enjoying each moment in time and achieving a state of thoughtless awareness, where the excessive stress-producing activities of the mind are neutralised without reducing alertness and effectiveness.

Meditation affects the body in exactly the opposite way that stress does, restoring it to a calm state and helping the body repair itself. It has proven to be very beneficial during menopause, helping to control many of the symptoms.

When practicing meditation your heart rate and breathing slow down, your blood pressure normalises and you use oxygen more efficiently through your breathing exercises, making it effective in short-term stress reduction and long-term health benefits. Scientific studies have revealed that the effects of meditation last well beyond the meditation session itself. In experienced meditators it seems the brain becomes persistently more active in the 'left prefrontal cortex', sitting just beneath the skull above the left eye. This brain region is associated with feeling good and with concentration and planning. Although scientists have used scanning equipment to discover this activity, they still do not fully understand why this occurs, but it does seem that meditating really can make you happy and more alert. This heightened pre-frontal activity is also what seems to tame the mind, giving you the power to deliberately keep your attention where you want it, though this will require some practice.

Benefits of Meditation

There are many benefits of meditating during menopause and it can bring about several positive feelings and thoughts in your mind and body.

Physiological Benefits

*Helps to increase blood flow and slows the heart rate, which will lower oxygen consumption. This is beneficial for those who suffer from high blood pressure.
*Decreases muscle tension so you feel more energetic and less fatigued.
*Helps to relax the nervous system, bringing about a deeper level of physical relaxation and helps to reduce anxiety attacks.
*Helps cure headaches and migraines.
*Can help stop smoking, drinking or drug addiction.

Psychological Benefits

*Can help build self-confidence by controlling your thoughts, giving you the ability to face your fears or phobias.
*Increases brain wave coherence, improves learning ability and memory.
*By learning to be less aggressive through control, you can improve relationships at work and at home.
*Encourages greater tolerance and composure and a well-balanced personality.
*Can help to reduce the dependency on pharmaceuticals and drugs and improve sleeping problems.
*Helps to develop an emotional maturity that will in turn help to ignore petty issues.

Spiritual Benefits

*Helps to balance the mind, body and soul and foster a deeper level of spiritual relaxation.
*Encourages a deeper understanding of yourself.
*Helps to keep things in perspective and provides a peace of mind, a

sense of happiness and increased compassion.
*Enables you to discover your purpose with an increased self-actualisation.
*Can help you to grow in wisdom and be forgiving towards others.
*Can change your attitude towards life.

Meditation Techniques

Most people find it difficult to meditate at the beginning. When you start to meditate you are entering a totally different dimension of reality. Normally in life we put a great deal of time and effort into achieving things, and there is probably a lot of struggle involved. Whereas meditation is the opposite of how we normally operate, so it will be hard to switch off from all the activities running around in your mind. Even when there are no distractions the mind will resist focus; it will want to keep chatting away to you, reminding you of things that need to be done. You will tell your mind to be still, but it won't want to be, it will bounce from one thought to the next, from images, to an idea, to different thoughts, everywhere, apart from where you want to focus.

So, when you start to meditate don't be too surprised if your mind won't co-operate. And don't get too frustrated, just keep practicing and eventually you will have some sort of control over it.

In fact, before you even begin to learn any meditation skills, I would recommend just sitting quietly somewhere, your body still, your speech silent, and your mind at ease. Allow your thoughts to come and go without trying to have any control over them at this stage. For now just allow them to drift into your mind and drift out again, without paying too much attention to them or analysing them too much. Don't question them, just let them be. If you feel you need to do something, then concentrate on your breathing. This is a very simple process of being mindful.

Once you are comfortable with this relaxation technique and not being too confrontational with your thoughts, you can try the next stage of developing your skills of concentration and focus.

For this I would recommend using your daily activities as a way to begin controlling your thoughts. Spend a few moments each day, when you are doing a particular activity, and concentrate on that moment in time, whether it is walking the dog, sending an e-mail or doing the housework. The point is, not to let your mind wander, just concentrate on the here and now, pay sole attention to what you are doing and block out all other thoughts. Listen to the sound of the keyboard as you type your e-mail, or feel the soles of your feet touch the ground as you walk. Concentrate only on what you are doing and don't allow any other thoughts to come into your mind. Hopefully, each day you will be able to control it for a little longer without any interruptions, and when you are confident that you have gained some control over your mind you can move into a more structured meditation routine.

Once you feel ready to start that routine, I suggest you begin by meditating for 15 minutes each day. Mornings are a good time, while the world is still dark, or the sun's just beginning to dawn, your mind is biologically programmed to be still. Obviously this won't be suitable for everyone, especially if you work irregular hours. Meditation has to fit into your routine. Whether you choose morning, afternoon or evening, it is beneficial to meditate at the same time each day if possible, especially when you are first learning, as this prepares your mind, body and spirit to be in a meditative state during that time. Just as lunchtime brings inspiration to eat, meditation time can bring inspiration to meditate. Your mind is a creature of habit, so use that tendency for your benefit.

As you become more professional at meditating you will be able to do it anywhere, anytime for a quick fix.

For The Beginner

Psychologically preparing yourself to meditate may make you more receptive to achieving success. You may want to use a special set of clothes just for meditation. Meditating in the same clothes can actively help, because when you meditate the energy in and around your body becomes more spiritualised, concentrated and powerful and can permeate the clothes you wear. This may help you to glide more smoothly into meditation next time.

Setting the Scene

If you have the space it's a good idea to set aside a room, corner or even a shelf where only meditation takes place. Your own spiritual energy accumulates in that area, making it easier for you to meditate. You may wish to light a candle. Watching a lighted candle can be an aid to meditation, looking at the flame may help to concentrate your mind. Incense will also help calm the chattering thoughts in your mind and focus the senses, or alternatively, mixtures of fragrant oils, herbs and spices can be prepared.

Breathing Techniques

Focusing on your breathing will help to calm the mind.
When you have cleared your mind of all thoughts, the breath is the last thing you will be aware of.
Try and keep your breathing at a constant pace and with total focus take three slow, deep breaths. Use a count of eight for your inhalation, then holdyour breath for a count of eight and exhale for the same. This keeps your breathing even and also gives you an oxygen boost, which relaxes you even further. After three breaths you will find your breathing is noticeably slower. Try to breathe in through your nose and out through your mouth.
When your mind wanders, which it inevitably will, just re-direct it and focus on the sound of your breathing; try and follow your breath with your mind as it enters and leaves your body.

Alternatively, you may benefit from using a mantra. This is the repetition of a sacred word or even just a word you like. Ommm is a very common mantra - it is said to be the vibrating sound of the universe. Whatever word you choose, the point of it is to force the mind to focus on a single thought.
Mala beads may also help your concentration. A mala is a string of 108 beads with one bead as the summit bead called a 'sumeru'. This is a tool used to keep your mind on the meditation practice. Malas are generally made from different materials such as tulsi, (basi) wood, sandal wood, or crystal. Each type of material has certain properties which subtly affect your subconscious mind.

Common Problems with Meditating

Can't Quiet the Mind
Many people find it difficult to calm the mind and stop the constant chatter of things to do and people to see, resulting in your thought patterns going down a different trail. The more you try to focus the more your mind betrays you.

Lack of Focus
Slightly different from not being able to quiet the mind - in as much as you are trying to focus on a specific idea, image sound or concept and you can't maintain that focal point.

Getting Distracted
This happens when you allow the sounds and noises of others to interrupt the time you have set aside for yourself. You need to be able to develop this skill in order to have strong meditation skills.

Finding the Time
There is no doubt that the world today seems a far busier place. The pace of life is hectic and our days seem to pass in a whirl of commitments - but we must prioritise and take the time to do things that improve our life.

Re-Cap
The first step is to decide that now is the right time for you to learn to meditate otherwise it won't work.

You really have to want to do it. Be prepared to practice and be patient with yourself in learning this new skill.

Choose your time, preferably the same time each day.

Choose the length of time for meditation.

Prepare your meditation area and wear your meditation clothes if you wish.

Start your meditation session by giving a blessing for the day - stating your hopes for the day ahead, or maybe a prayer - it's your choice. The purpose is to prepare your mind for meditation.

Sit with a straight back. Don't try to meditate lying down because you may fall asleep. Meditation brings relaxation and peace but at the same time this is a dynamic peace and our sense of awareness is heightened. Afterwards you will have a positive feeling for the world and a renewed sense of dynamism.

Don't eat before meditating. Your body will be lethargic with digestion after a heavy meal.

It is not necessary to meditate in the lotus posture, it is fine to do it in a chair as long as the back is straight.

You may like to take a shower before meditating.

Once you have mastered the 'single thought' technique - which may take a while - you can proceed to the next stage of 'no thought at all'. Achieving this 'silent mind' is difficult but a powerful experience. When a thought appears, try to view it as separate from yourself and make a conscious effort to throw it out of your mind. Not an easy task, don't get discouraged, just keep practicing and you will eventually attain the power to control your thoughts and on occasion stop them completely.

There is a wealth of information out there on meditation. This is just a small insight into something that may improve the quality of your life. If you would like more information or to develop the skill further, you might like to take a look at
www.how-to-meditate.org
www.successconsciousness.com
www.eckharttolle.com

Enlightenment

Enlightenment is a word that has many different applications - I will merely try to give you an introduction and allow you to explore and expand your knowledge on the subject yourself.

Mindfulness and meditation may help lead to seeing things clearer and finding enlightenment.
By being mindful of yourself, you take the time to look at things and see them and appreciate them for their true being. For example each new day begins with a one of a kind sunrise, which should be appreciated for its beauty. But for most people, it is viewed as the start of another day. Time to get up, organise the family, have breakfast, go to work and so on.
By taking it for granted you have lacked awareness and miss out on its beauty.

An enlightened person may go through the same situations as a non-enlightened person, but her awareness has shifted to a higher perspective where she sees the divine in every event, person and experience.

In life there are too many things most of us take for granted most of the time. Like the love of our family and friends, or the roof over our heads, or that we are not in some form of extreme pain.
The unfortunate thing is that most of us don't appreciate the things we have until we lose them. Only if we go blind do we start to think it was so nice when we could see, only when we have an illness do we appreciate having good health.

When we are mindful we are more appreciative of what we have, when we have it, which will in turn make us feel much happier.

Being mindful also gives you the strength to deal with distress. When something happens, or someone says or does something, we react with either anger, or happiness, or hatred. By being aware and mindful you are fully responsible and in control of how you feel. For example, if you are in a situation where you are feeling ' he makes me feel so angry' - think about the fact that if you were in a room with 10 other people in the same situation, not all of them would be angry, but they would react in different ways. You are the one who is angry about the situation, so it is correct to say YOU feel angry about what he said instead of HE makes you angry. The important difference here is you are taking full responsibility for your own feelings rather than putting the responsibility on someone else. You have become aware of who you are and you are more mindful of your reaction, whether it is anger, hatred or disappointment. You will now be able to dispel the feeling and no longer be a slave to your emotions and reactions. Instead you have developed a say over how you should feel. To put it simply, you will feel more content and in control of yourself.

When you understand this, you will have a feeling of awareness with everything around you, and you will have let go of who you thought you were, so that you can paradoxically become the person you have always been.

Create A Sacred Space

Whether it's for religious, spiritual, personal reasons or meditation , creating a personal altar in your home can be a beautiful inspiring place, where you can focus your thoughts, inspirations and desires. It's a place where you can give thanks, prayers, offerings and blessings or honour and remember loved ones.
In many parts of the world a small altar is a traditional part of the home, where the spiritual world reaches into the world of the every day.

There are no rules to follow when creating your own personal altar. It can be just for you alone or to share with family and friends.

Create it from your inner thoughts and change and develop it as you wish.
When you create your altar or mini temple, whether it's an elaborate structure or a small shelf in a corner, it will be a place to centre and renew yourself, a place to nourish your soul and restore your sense of the sacred.

Use objects that hold meaning for you in the altar you have created. These items may be statues, paintings, photos, candles, flowers, oils and incense, crystals or gems, and whatever other personal or symbolic objects help to open your heart and focus your mind.

Types of Altars:

Religious Altars
For prayer and communicating with your God. As well as candles and incense you will probably include icons, spiritual images and objects that represent your particular belief system. Their presence being reminders of the symbolic ideas for which they stand and a way to communicate on a tangible and personal level with God.

Memorial Altar - Alter for a loved one.
This will be a very personal altar which you will create from the love you had for this person, or it may even be for a beloved family pet. Personal objects and photographs which hold special memories will probably take pride of place, maybe alongside a vase of favourite flowers, candles and incense.
All of the objects you bring to this altar are to help you focus spiritually and to remember the loved one in life. It is important to choose items that remind you of your whole relationship with them, not just the end of their life. The shrine will also act as a focus for all the thoughts and emotions you still need to communicate to the person who is lost.

Meditation Altar
A meditation altar can be as simple as a candle or an object to focus on, or you might like to embellish it further by adding a miniature Zen garden. This is another popular way to focus the mind for meditation. The serenity of a Zen garden has an almost hypnotic effect and taking time with your designs will help the mind become relaxed and centred. You can buy these Zen gardens complete or you may decide to make your own with some sand and pebbles, maybe adding fresh flowers to represent living and natural forms. Use chopsticks or a small rake/comb to create spirals and circles in the sand and around the stones and flowers. When you have created a pattern that comes from your inner consciousness, sit back and

contemplate it. Empty your mind of its clutter and absorb the simplicity and peace of the natural forms in front of you.

Tip – This is a great calming activity for the grandchildren as well. Give them their own shallow bowl or tray with some sand, flowers and pebbles and let them create their very own Zen garden. It will help to quiet their frustrations in their busy little world.

Alters and sacred places do not only have to be religious or spiritual, you can create them for such things as:

Motivation
Motivation comes with feeling self-directed and hopeful. Setting yourself a goal is motivating in itself. Just make sure you set goals that are achievable but still stretch your capabilities. Making an altar for motivation is a positive statement and will encourage you to move forward.
Your altar should sparkle with energy and light. Place it in a sunny position so it catches the light. Choose a beautiful shimmering piece of fabric to use as an alter cloth and decorate with your favourite flowers. Use yellow candles to help you concentrate on your goals and burn uplifting oil such as bergamot, geranium and orange. Listening to music can also be a great motivator.
While sitting at your alter review your achievements of the previous day, and write a list of your goals for the day ahead and re-confirm you long term goals.

A New Beginning
May mean starting a new chapter in your life - the menopause being the perfect opportunity. Whatever the new beginning is, there will be encounters and opportunities that will shape your future.
Like the 'motivation altar' try and place it so it will be bathed in sunshine. Add a vase of flowers to symbolise new growth and natural energy. Burn white candles which represent new beginnings. Place a small bell on your altar and ring it three times at the beginning of your ritual; this will help to call new realities into your life and focus on your hopes and wishes for the future.

Burn an incense mixture of:
2 parts dried rosemary, 1 part dried thyme 1 part dried lemongrass; add a few drops of rosemary essential oil.
Pound the dry ingredients together using a pestle and mortar and add an essential oil. Mix in well with finger tips. Burn a few pinches of incense on the altar using a small incense burner.

Creativity and Inspiration
Is the energy you put into everything you create and it flows through us all. An altar reflecting this energy can be inspirational and a place to tune into the creative spirit.
In this special place you have created, you can leave behind the limitations of self-consciousness and open your mind to new ideas, try out your dreams and nourish your imagination.
Make your altar vibrant and full of colour, let your imagination go wild and dress it with flamboyance and confidence to express your personality and creativity.

Colour Associations for Candles

White - Spiritual enlightenment, healing, peace and purity
Yellow - Intelligence, communication, concentration, movement
Orange - Attraction, stimulation, strength, luck
Gold - Understanding, confidence, prosperity, cosmic influences
Pink - Harmony, nurturing, family, affection
Red - Energy, life, courage, passion
Violet - Spirituality, inner harmony, wisdom
Purple - Spirituality, inner harmony, wisdom
Indigo - Cleansing, meditation
Blue - Wisdom, inspiration, truth, healing
Green - Love, nature, renewal, abundance
Brown - Home, wealth, stability
Silver - Secrets, compromise
Grey - Secrets, compromise
Black - Conclusions, banishes guilt, regret and negativity

Incense Associations

Frangipani - Blessing of love and friendships
Frankincense - Cleansing and blessing, banishing bad influences and enhancing insight
Honeysuckle - For healing and psychic power
Jasmine - Increasing sensitivity and to bless meditation
Lotus - Clearing the mind
Musk - For courage and vitality
Myrrh - Purifying and cleansing of negative thoughts
Patchouli - Grounding, fertility, protection and prosperity
Pine - Strength and reversal of negative energy
Rose - Emotional healing and expression of feelings
Sandalwood - Protection, healing, and granting of wishes
Vanilla - Rejuvenation, love and mental concentration
White sage - Purifying and cleansing sacred space

Dharma

Dharma comes from the Sanskrit word 'dhr' meaning to 'uphold' or to 'sustain'.

In Buddhism Dharma refers to the collective teachings of the Buddha, and in Hinduism it is associated with a system of guidelines for one to follow in life such as the right way of living, proper conduct, duty or righteousness.

In the Western world Dharma translates into the way you are meant to live. It is what you were born to be, and it is the path of life on which you will achieve the greatest degree of happiness, success and fulfilment.

Dharma is like wearing a pair of comfortable shoes. You feel good in them because they fit you so well. When you are out of dharma and you find yourself off your intended path, it's like wearing a pair of shoes which are too tight, too restricting and uncomfortable, and you feel miserable wearing them.
When you are in dharma all of your talents and energy emerge and

converge to produce positive effects for you and all of those around you. You can't help but exude qualities of passion, peace, happiness and fulfilment. As a result you will naturally practice patience, honesty, compassion, self-control, forgiveness and reason. Likewise, living in your dharma will also help you let go of unnecessary anger, resentment, judgment, envy, greed and jealousy. You and everyone around you benefit from your dharma.

Many people live their entire lives without being in dharma or on their intended path. There is absolutely no joy in this. To live the greatest life you are capable of living you need to know who you are and where you are going. This is your life and it is your responsibility to make it the best you possibly can.
So take a moment to think about your dharma shoes, are they comfortable and fit just right or are they too tight or too loose?

More information about Dharma can be found at
www.aboutdharma.org

Karma

The word is Sanskrit and means act, action or deed and refers to the fact that humans determine their own destinies through the qualities of their acts. Man is master of his own fate. A person is not born great or small, it is his karma that makes him noble or criminal.

Karma is created through body, speech and mind. It's what we intentionally do, say and think. If we act without any intention no karma is created.

Watch your thoughts for they become words
Watch your words for they become actions
Watch your actions for they become habits
Watch your habits for they become your character
Watch your character for it becomes your destiny

Words of Inspiration

Read uplifting words for a positive feeling and reading them before you go to sleep may help give you good dreams , so you will wake in a bright mood.

Bless your day - when you wake, before you even get out of bed, take a moment to offer gratitude for the day ahead, smile and hope it will be a successful one.

Surround yourself with positive feelings and with things that inspire and uplift you. Place photographs or pictures on your desk that are meaningful for you. Choose objects that inspire you and smells that uplift your senses. Your subconscious mind will absorb all of this information even when you are not fully aware of your surroundings and will give you a feeling of general well-being.

As you are about to put the letter into the post box or hit the send button - stop for a moment and offer your good wishes or thanks, or whatever special thought relates to the correspondence for a positive outcome and then carry on.

Be friendly to people around you, be courteous and polite, and make an effort to connect with them. Find joy in greeting others and treat them with genuine respect and appreciation. Hopefully your response will be reciprocated, surrounding you with a positive uplifting atmosphere, bringing about a sense of well-being.

Create a sense of good feeling by lighting candles, burning fragrant incense, or even feeding the birds.

Have a dream or a goal - something to look forward to or to aim for. Just make sure that it's what you really want because you might just get it!

Think good thoughts and look at events in your life with a positive eye. This will enhance the good times and soften the difficult times.

Keep your word – respect yourself and your promises. If you give your word you should do your very best to keep it. Don't make promises you can't keep.

Good sense of humour – Laughter is the wine of the soul and laughing with pure delight is something we should do often. With a good sense of humour you can laugh when you're happy and can even laugh when you cry. Humour is a great friend on your life's journey.

HOLISTIC HEALING

Holistic healing treats the person as a whole and believes there is a communication between mind and body.

Ayurveda

The Ayurveda concept is a 5000 year old traditional Indian medical system that balances and integrates mind, body and spirit. Which means that it is holistic and based on the principal that disease is the natural end result of living out of harmony with our environment. Ayurveda's approach to healing is to re-establish harmony between self and environment.

Ayurveda views every person as different, with unique life situations and mind/body concepts. Your uniqueness determines a lot about you, your personality and your body. Understanding them will help you to know how to heal yourself in order to be totally healthy.

According to Ayurveda concepts, everyone has five basic elements which are: space, fire, water, air and earth.

These elements combine with each other to produce three Ayurveda body types called 'Dosha's'.

There are three dosha's that everyone is made up of, but it is the dominant one or two that comprise a person's mind-set. Dominance of the three dosha's will shift with age, time of day or night and seasons.

Dosha's relate closely to the basic elements of nature and to specific functions of the body. Balance of these dosha's is thought to be required for optimum health. Ayurveda stresses proper diet for maintaining good health and treating disease. Herbal remedies are prescribed based upon the person's diet.

The Three Dosha Types Are:

Vata = Air and Space - tend to be of a small thin build
Pitta = Fire and Water - body type is more of a medium build
Kapha= Water and Earth - appearance is usually bigger and well developed

Vata Dosha - initiates all forms of activity and motion in the body. It acts as a network of communication from tissue to tissue and cell to cell. It is responsible for perception, assimilation and reaction.

Pitta Dosha - responsible for all types of transformations in the body. Pitta controls digestion of food, and is associated with the chemical reaction and changes taking place in the body. This dosha also controls emotions like anger, fear and boldness and is responsible for hunger, appetite and thirst. The functions of pitta are more physical compared to vata.

Kapha Dosha - is the third important part of dosha. This dosha is the cohesive energy in the body, smooth's out problems and provides support when needed.

To find out your dosha type and more information on Ayurveda visit:

www.chopra.com
www.ayurveda.com
www.ayurvediccenter.com

Aura

Your aura, also known as the Human Energy Field (HEF), is the manifestation of universal energy around the human body, and consists of seven layers which resonate at a higher vibration than the physical body. This multi coloured mist of vital energy radiates through you and around you.

Etheric layer: Bright in a healthy person, pale in the ailing
Emotional Layer: Used as a store house for emotions
Mental Layer: A weak mental layer indicates lack of will power
Astral Layer: Deals with matters of the heart, provides links between body, mind and spirit
Etheric Template: Energy field of communication and creative expression
Celestial Layer: Represents visual senses
Ketheric Layer: When shining bright indicates a mind unafraid of judgment or criticism

Although the aura is generally a mixture of various colours, every aura has a distinctive shade:

Blue: Peaceful, content, for seekers on spiritual paths
Green: Ambitious with tendencies to achieve
White; Eccentric and bored with the mundane, chameleon type personality
Orange: Creatively communicative
Red; Living life in the fast lane and fighting for convictions
Purple: Inclination towards magic, strong psychic abilities

Aura Cleansing Exercise:
Shower or bathe in Epsom salts and take deep cleansing breaths.

Chakras

Chakra is another word that has its origins in Sanskrit and means 'wheel of light'.

Chakras are part of the subtle energy system and are like personal energy centres in the body, spinning like a wheel or a vortex. Positioned along the spine, the chakras are linked to each other and also link the body to its aura.

Each chakra has its own frequency and vibration through which energy is received and transmitted. They symbolise the connection between the spiritual and the physical, and coincide with the body's endocrine system (which is the system of glands that secrete hormones into the bloodstream to regulate the body).

There are seven main chakras in the body and different parts of the body are associated with each chakra. Each has its own associated colour.

Colour	Endocrine Gland	Area of body governed
Red	Adrenals	Spinal column, kidneys
Orange	Gonads	Reproductive system
Yellow	Pancreas	Stomach, liver, gall bladder, reproductive system
Green	Thymus	Heart, blood, vagus nerve, circulatory system
Blue	Thyroid	Bronchial, vocal apparatus, lungs, alimentary canal
Indigo	Pituitary	Lower brain, left eye, ears, nose, nervous system
Violet/white	Pineal	Upper brain, right eye

Chakras may become out of balance, which means they might be blocked, or be too open, or spinning too fast or too slow. This might be caused by stress or emotional issues. When they are unbalanced, various mental, emotional and psychological conditions may occur. There are various ways of balancing chakras, including sound, colour, yoga, crystal and spiritual healing

A healer trained in manipulating the energy flow can assist you in getting misaligned chakras back to functioning properly. It may take one or more sessions to get you energy levels up to par. Afterwards there are a variety of healthy actions you can take to help keep them open, allowing your energy to flow naturally.

Psychological Function of the Chakras

Base Chakra	Sex, procreation, vitality, creativity
Sacral Chakra	Power, identity, status, aggression
Solar Plexus Chakra	Energy, emotions
Heart Chakra	Love, love of self, universal love, devotion, compassion
Throat Chakra	Speech, understanding, truth
Head Chakra	Focus, knowledge
Crown Chakra	Inspiration, Surrender to consciousness

Incantations

To help balance and align your chakra energy repeat each of the incantations listed below. Speak the first part of the phrase out loud as you inhale and the second part of the phrase as you exhale. Repeat each one 10 times and when you are finished you will feel centred and balanced:

Incantations

Inhale	Exhale
My Energy	Free of blockages
My Root Chakra	Is deeply grounded
My Sacral Chakra Juices	Are creative and bold
My Solar Plexus	Feels mellow and calm
My Heart	Is filled with love
My Throat	Speaks the truth
My Head	Intuits inner knowledge
My Crown	Projects inspiration
My Chakras	Are spinning in alignment
My Aura	Is colourful and bright
My Light Body	Beams Brightly
I am	Centred and balanced

Drumming

Drumming activates the heart chakra, balancing the descending higher chakra energies against the ascending lower chakra frequencies. Research is now verifying the therapeutic effects of ancient rhythmic drumming techniques. Drumming accelerates physical healing, boosts the immune system and produces a feeling of well-being.

Chakracise

Strengthen and balance your chakras through exercise:

Base Chakra - Stomping your feet upon the ground, marching, doing squats

Sacral Chakra - Pelvic thrusts and circular pelvis movement

Solar Plexus Chakra - Dancing, belly dancing, the twist, hula hooping

Head Chakra - Push-ups, swimming (breast stroke) and hugging yourself

Throat Chakra - Gargle with salt water, sing or scream

Head Chakra - Visualisation, remote viewing and lucid dreaming

Crown Chakra - Exercise through meditation or prayer

Sensuous Living

Is about being aware of those sensory moments that we know give us pleasure. Unfortunately, in this fast-paced life, many of us have had our senses dulled by overstimulation and neglect. We are constantly bombarded with huge arrays of sounds, smells and visual images. Our senses are so over-stimulated that we automatically block out sensations in order to survive. We have become so hardened by daily stress we have lost the ability to relax into sensual joy. We have stopped appreciating how much our senses add, not only to our sexual pleasure, but also to our quality of life on a daily basis. We have grown empty and cold through our pre-occupation with money and achievement.

Most of us are starved of positive sensations, soothing sounds to relax us, tastes and smells that satisfy us, the simple beauty of nature and the sensuality of being touched and caressed.

We need to re-awaken our senses and delight in the five physical senses of touch, sight, hearing, smell and taste. Indulge yourself and fill your environment with beautiful objects and sensory experiences. Play music you love and take the time to really hear it. Burn aromatherapy oils and notice the depth of the aroma they produce; eat your favourite food and taste the wonderful flavours it has; walk barefoot in the grass and be aware of how it feels against your feet, and really see what you are looking at. Take the time to absorb the beauty of what's in front of you. By being mindful of all of your senses, you will be reminded of a whole world that you had forgotten about.

Try closing your eyes while moisturising every part of your body with your favourite cream or lotion, be aware of your sense of touch and notice how your skin feels.

Try putting on some mellow music and dance slowly; dance to the beat of the background music. Really feel your body move and how you are in control of each movement you make.

Take a shower or bath in a darkened room, with just one small tea light candle. Enjoy the sensuality of your body and enjoy the moment.

Sensuality in The Bedroom

Sight: Experiment with lighting in the bedroom. Having a bright light on will probably be too harsh and not very romantic or very flattering. On the other hand, no light at all will dull your other senses and not give you the opportunity to become aroused by your partners naked body. Try different types of lighting, such as coloured bulbs or scarves placed over lamps to create subtle shades of colour, and of course, candles will always create a romantic atmosphere. Looking into each other's eyes as you make love will maximise your sensual pleasure. Hang mirrors in your room or strategically place one in your wardrobe and leave the door open. You and your partner may find it highly erotic to catch sight of yourselves during love making, and wearing sexy lingerie or underwear is always a visual turn on.

Hearing: Music can be particularly powerful in affecting your moods. Choose music that you both enjoy and will stir up passionate feelings or remind you of when you were first together. You could also experiment with different types of music; make some time together to listen to various types of sounds. You might be surprised to learn that the sounds of African drum music or the natural sounds of nature have an effect on you. Apart from listening to music, make sure you express your feelings to each other. Make some noise if your lover is touching you in an especially pleasurable way, and allow yourself to respond with moans of enjoyment, giving encouragement to carry on.

Smell: Is the most evocative of our senses and can be very powerful in changing moods and bringing back memories. We each have our own 'personal scent', just as we have unique fingerprints, with no two being the same.
Women tend to have a sharper sense of smell, especially when ovulating. Some women find the smell of a man's sweaty body

offensive, while others find they are aroused by it. Scents that are similar to a man's sexual musk can also be highly arousing to women. Men tend to act negatively towards artificial scents, especially when sprayed freely around the house. Natural oils and room sprays would be far more suitable. You can heighten your awareness of smell by paying attention to how your partner smells throughout the day. Take notice of how he smells after his morning shower and how he smells when he comes home in the evening. Pay attention to any reaction you have to certain smells. Is the clean fresh morning smell more appealing to you than the smell after a hard day at work, and do certain fragrances or aftershaves elicit strong memories? Choose your aromas carefully and don't make the mistake of smothering yourself in perfume. You don't want to drown out your pheromones, which are the natural smell we produce during sex and what we are attracted to.

Touch: When you are with your partner try and focus your attention on the sense of touch - stay in your body instead of in your head. By this I mean don't let your mind wander off into some fantasy; pay attention to how it feels when you are kissing your partner. Focus on how your lips feel against theirs, pay attention to the feel of their tongue as it plays with yours and how it makes your body feel. If your partner is caressing you, stay in the moment and notice how the touch feels on your body. Really feel the sensation, and follow the movement of their hands on your skin. If you are caressing your partner, concentrate on your hands touching their skin and the sensation you are experiencing. Don't allow your mind to drift off, focus and concentrate on what you are doing and take pleasure and enjoyment from the moment.

Taste: The main organ responsible for taste is our tongue, and although there are many taste receptors situated on the taste buds, there are just four different types of receptors that are responsible for the thousands of flavours we taste each day, sweet, sour, salty and bitter. Many of us are guilty of eating without appreciating the taste of our food; it's merely fuel for our body, which is sad because food is so much more. By having the ability to really taste the flavours and enjoy the textures, we could gain so much more pleasure and enjoyment from nourishing our bodies with food. Learn to preserve your sense of taste by taking time to chew your food and fully experience the taste. Draw a small amount of air into your mouth while chewing your food to increase the rate at which aromas ascend towards your nasal cavity. Try different types of food with various spices and flavours. Instead of salt, try enhancing your food with fresh and fragrant herbs and spices. This will keep your olfactory nerves from getting bored. Try different combinations to excite your taste buds (and your partners), like ice cold water with slices of lemon and frozen grapes, or sweet white wine with dark chocolate, or red wine with fresh figs and roasted almonds, or iced tea with fresh mint, sliced green apple and sharp cheddar cheese. Blindfold your partner and feed him a selection of foods. Make it fun and choose things that are sweet, salty, sour and bitter. Try things like small portions of bananas, chocolate, honey orange slices, lemon slices, ice cream, and whipped cream. The taste of your lover's body can also be a pleasurable experience, nibbling, licking and tasting your partner will certainly enhance your lovemaking. Try some of the edible lotion and potion recipes we have included as an aperitif, before moving on to the main course!!

Tantric Sex

Tantric sex or Tantra as it's often known can be inspiring and bring new life and depth into your lovemaking.

Tantric sex is about consciousness. We have, over time, developed into creatures of habit. We make love in the same way, same position and probably on the same days of the week. For most people sex is all about achieving the end goal of 'the orgasm'. We get so lost in the rush to get there that we forget the pleasure of the journey. If we stopped being so concerned about reaching that end goal, we could be more involved with our partner and enjoy the intimacy and pleasure on a much deeper level. After all, how intimate can you really be when you're having sex with the lights off or your eyes closed and you're lost in some fantasy. How connected to your partner are you in those moments? Fantasies are fine if they involve both of you and they can certainly enhance your love making, just get the balance right.

Tantric sex encourages lust, not only in a sexual sense, but lust for life, full of sensual living and feeling. This includes the delicious taste of food and drink, exploring flavours and textures, beautiful music, flowers and exercise.

www.tantric-sex.org www.templeoftantra.com

Just The Two of You

Set aside an evening once in a while and have a special night in with your partner.

Prepare a Romantic Bath
Transform your bathroom into a fantasy setting for your romantic bath together. Dim the lights, if possible, use candles of varying sizes on counter tops to set the scene, fill the bath with bubbles or you may prefer bath milks, exotic oils or infused mineral salts. Whatever gives you the most pleasure. Sprinkle a few fresh rose petals over the floor and a few in the bath itself. Fill the bathroom with exotic aromas, burn oils or incense along with your candles and play romantic music. Place a small table by the side of the bathtub and set with some sensual foods such as chocolate-covered strawberries and champagne, or try making a cocktail with a chocolate liqueur base and sip with a bowl of fresh raspberries. Choose foods that are easy and fun to eat and that you will both enjoy. Have plenty of freshly laundered bath towels and robes ready for when you get out.
Besides eating and drinking together, washing each other is sure to be a romantic endeavour; use soft cloths, sponges or loofahs with luxurious smelling soaps or body wash to create a rich lather. Fill a jug with the warm-scented bath water and slowly pour it over your partner, repeat the process as often as you like - it feels wonderful.

Bath Oil Recipe
2 drops Neroli essential oil

1 drop Rose essential oil
2 drops Ylang Ylang essential oil
Mix together and add to the bath just before getting in, so the oils don't vaporise

Top 10 Sexiest Essential Oils

Make sure you use pure essential oils rather than fragranced oils, as these are made with chemicals rather than the pure essence of the flower, they could irritate the skin, and the smell will also be far inferior.

1. Ylang Ylang- Sensual and exotic, good balance between feminine and masculine scents
2. Sandalwood - Relaxing and sensual with sweet woody notes
3. Jasmine - Enchanting, rich tropical scent
4. Neroli - Soothing, floral aroma
5. Rose - Luxurious oil with soothing properties
6. Mandarin - Delicate scent which is soothing and uplifting
7. Clary sage - Sweet and musky
8. Lavender - Will help relax you and your partner and ease anxiety
9. Ginger - Warm and sexy to help spice up your mood
10. Patchouli - Warm and rich with sweet, spicy, woody notes

There are many sensuous oils out there to try, and creating your own mood scents depends on what you like. Familiarise yourself with some of them to see which ones you prefer and then you can make up your own signature scent to use in massage oils, room sprays, burning oils, bath oil - whatever takes your fancy.

*Choose scented candles, incense or oils with care, ones that are too flora for example may be off putting.

Massage – The Dance of Love

A sensual massage is a great way to build intimacy and closeness with your partner.

• Start by massaging your partners face and head. No need to use oils when you do this part as it won't feel particularly good. Sit crossed legged and have your partner put their head in your lap (face up). Run your fingers several times through your loved ones hair, from the base of his neck to the top of his head. Massage the temples in circles, grasp large chunks of hair close to the roots and tug gently. Using your fingertips, lightly stroke the forehead, starting at the centre and moving towards the temples. Stroke from the centre of the nose, across the cheeks and out towards the ears. Tease your partner's lips with a fingertip.

• Have your partner lie face down, warm your hands by rubbing them together, lubricate with a massage oil or lubricant of your choice. Begin at the neck, using thumbs to knead the neck and upper back, work across one shoulder and down the arm, wrap your hand around the upper arm and use a twisting motion to massage down the length of the arm. Use fingertips to stoke the back of the hand. Using your thumb, make circles in their palm, interlace your fingers with theirs and squeeze, gently rock their fingers back and forth, stroking each from base to tip. Work back up their arm, across their back to the other side and repeat.

• Lightly drag fingers from the backs of their hands, up the arms and across the shoulders to meet in the centre of the back. The touch should be feather soft but shouldn't tickle.

• Place your hand in the small of your partner's back and stroke up and down, one hand on each side. Use firm but gentle pressure and don't work directly over the spine. Kneed the flesh around your partners neck, start gently and gradually get firmer around the area where muscles are tense. Be careful not to pinch, then return to the long effleurage strokes you started with.

• Next, starting at the lower back, use both hands to rub the flesh at the side of the torso, gently pushing up and away from the spine, slowly move up towards the head. When you reach the neck, sweep your hands down to the lower back and repeat three or four times. Use thumbs to make small circular movements and slowly move up either side of the spine. Sweep hands down either side of the torso and repeat two or three times and then gradually work down to your partner's buttocks.

• Knead the back of one of your partner's legs, starting just below the buttocks and working all the way down the leg; be careful on the back of the knee (this is a very ticklish spot for some). Press with fingertips all around the ankle, move the foot back and forth in circles. Grasp the foot with both hands. The fingers should be on the top side of the foot, the thumbs on the sole. Stroke firmly from heel to toe, make circles in the arch, bend toes gently upwards to give a good stretch, run fingers up the leg, across the buttocks and lower back and to the opposite side. Repeat for other leg.

• Ask your partner to turn over, straddle them and massage their arms and hands again from the front. Now is a good time to teasingly kiss their eyelids, cheeks, lips and neck.

• Rub the chest and stomach using light feathery strokes. Be careful not to push too hard, it can be uncomfortable or even painful. Work down the sides and massage the sides of the hips - you can use a firmer touch here.

• As your hands move from the torso to the legs you will hit all kinds of erogenous zones. You can pretend to be very professional and pay no attention to their reaction - or you can give them a naughty smile and keep right on rubbing. Either way you will drive them crazy (in a good way). Massage their legs using the same techniques you used on the backs of the legs. The front of the shins can be very sensitive so use a lighter touch here.

• When the massage is finished you can go back over sensitive spots with a feathery touch to heighten their anticipation even more, or you can move right on to the 'Happy Ending'! Use your own special techniques here.

During the massage take some time every now and then to add extra stimulation into your massage movements, such as light feathery kisses, softly blowing or licking the skin.

Incorporating objects into your massage can also heighten the senses. Use things such as ice, feathers, fresh flowers, massage balls or anything that you think will help give a stimulating sensual massage.

Sexy Lotions and Potions Recipes

Sensual Massage Oil
4oz. grape seed oil
15 drops Rose oil
15 drops Ylang ylang oil

Mix essential oils together, adjust the amounts if necessary to suit your preference, add to grape seed oil, pour into small bottle and shake well.

Spicy Massage Oil
4 oz. carrier oil of choice (sweet almond, grape seed, apricot kernel oil)
15 drops sandalwood oil
9 drops cinnamon oil
6 drops peppermint oil
5 drops black pepper oil

Mix essential oils together as above

Edible Massage Lubricant
¼ cup glycerin (for heating effect)
¼ teaspoon honey
¼ teaspoon vanilla extract (clear not brown)
¼ teaspoon flavouring of choice (be careful of mint and cinnamon!) try chocolate, vanilla, coconut, orange
1 drop food colouring

Mix together well add flavouring and bottle. This lubricant is water soluble and will heat up when you blow on it.

Edible Massage Lubricant Two
¼ cup filtered water
¼ cup vegetable glycerin
1- 2 teaspoons vanilla or chocolate extract

Mix well together and bottle. Try different flavour combinations such as chocolate and mint (small amount), raspberry and vanilla, or chocolate and orange.

Edible Massage Oil
3 oz. sweet almond oil
2 oz. grape seed oil
1 oz. sunflower oil
1 teaspoon natural flavour oil of choice

Mix oils together and add flavour oil, adjust according to taste.

Edible Honey Dust Body Powder
8 oz. corn starch or arrow root powder
2 oz. honey powder
2 oz. vanilla powder

Mix well and sift into jar - Apply using fluffy feathers.

Edible Lotion Bars
If oils aren't your thing, try making this edible lotion bar - a solid bar of moisturising lotion which feels good and tastes great.

2 oz. beeswax
2 oz. coconut oil
1 oz. cocoa butter
1 - 2 tablespoons flavouring extract

Melt the beeswax on a low heat, add the coconut oil and cocoa butter. Remove from heat, add flavouring. Pour into moulds, such as ice cube trays. Let the mixture solidify and then pop out and let the massage begin.

Sin Tin Massage Candle
Try making this wonderful massage candle to heighten your partner's senses even further!

Massage candles are basically soy candles. Soy wax-melts at a lower temperature than paraffin wax, making it safe to use on the skin and quite soft. For massage candles, the wax must be a high-quality one that won't irritate your skin.

The soy wax is melted down and combined with oils and butters to allow it to be absorbed. Without these additions, the wax would cool and harden as it was being massaged into the skin.

The instructions are simple: light the candle, wait 10 to 15 minutes so there is a wax pool to draw from; blow out the candle if you wish and pour the warm wax onto your partner's body and begin the massage.

Recipe
3 oz. soy wax
1 oz. liquid oil (such as apricot kernel oil, sweet almond oil, jojoba or olive oil)
¼ oz. skin safe fragrance / essential oil
Candle wicks
Candle tin

Measure out all ingredients, melt soy wax in a double boiler or in microwave in short 30-second bursts. Add your chosen liquid oil and warm through. Remove from heat and add your fragrance. Stir and wait for the mixture to cool slightly before pouring into your candle tin or container; this will ensure you have a smooth surface on your candle. Place the wick in the centre of the tin and wait for the candle to harden. Once solid, trim the wick. You can now burn the candle and pour the moisturising warm wax over your partner and enjoy the consequences!

Sensual Linen Spray
This sensual linen spray contains oils that are both aphrodisiacs and relaxants, to give that extra added touch to your night time retreat.

20 drops sandalwood
10 drops rose oil
10 drops bergamot oil
6 drops ginger oil
6 drops lime oil

4 drops jasmine oil
4 drops ylang ylang oil
150ml Spray bottle
Distilled water

Fill spray bottle two thirds full with distilled water. In a bowl mix together all essential oils - adjust the amounts to suit your preference if needs be. Use a small funnel to pour essential oils into the bottle of water, screw on top and shake well. Place in the fridge for 24 hours to cure. The scent may change slightly once it has had time to sit. If you would like to add more of certain essentials oils now is the time to do it. Shake well and spray a light mist over your bed linens, towels, robes or any other fabrics you want to be lightly fragranced.

Friends

Start by knowing yourself, liking yourself and being your own best friend. Get to know yourself or remind yourself of whom you are. Now that you are entering this second phase of your life, it is the perfect time to get to know the new you.

Explore and understand your qualities including your strongest points and weakest . Be totally honest with yourself.

What motivates you?
How do you express yourself?
Take a look around and see what you have chosen to surround yourself with.

Look at the photos and paintings on your walls.
Are the objects around you representative of happy or sad times?
Do you like to wear comfortable or fashionable clothes?
What are your friends like? Supportive, trustworthy etc.
What books do you like to read? Drama, fiction, biographies, romance, non-fiction.
What kind of TV programmes do you like? Reality, news, drama, documentaries.
What kind of car do you drive? Impressive, reliable.

Observe how you react and respond in certain situations. How do you handle stress or criticism; do you get embarrassed easily? Do you like to be in control of situations or do you thrive on the unknown?

Ask yourself as many questions as you can think of to get to know yourself. This is not a quiz and there are no right or wrong answers. It is an exploration to help you become more self-aware, to really know and understand yourself, to be happy with who you are and to become your own best friend.

Most of us have traits or bad habits, or have done something we are not particularly proud of, but now is the time to begin to look at your-self with a more objective, kinder eye and grow beyond them.

- Be a nice person
- Mean what you say
- Help others
- Don't be too serious
- Respect yourself
- Appreciate everything in life
- Be loving
- Don't succumb to boredom, greed, or jealousy
- Be happy
- Have compassion
- Have fun
- Respect those who have given their lives
- Be kind
- Eat healthy food
- Be honest
- Don't indulge your senses too much
- Spend some time alone with your thoughts

"Friendship with oneself is all important because without it one cannot be friends with anyone else in the world" - *Eleanor Roosevelt*

Spending time with friends is one of the simplest things you can do to rev up the happiness stakes in your life.

Scientists at Harvard University found that happiness is catching. If you are friends with a positive person then 25 percent of their cheerfulness rubs off on you. But a friend is so much more - we need friends we can laugh with, cry with, have fun with, support, trust and love.

Healthy friendships are full of good feelings, you are able to be yourself. A good friend should build you up, not bring you down. Friends don't seek to serve their own needs, but rather seek to help others through encouragement, moral support and offering shoulders to cry on.
When we face difficult times in our lives good friends listen to our troubles and encourage us to face the next day.
Friends will respect your decisions whether they agree or not, but at the same time be able to share their concerns and opinions with you honestly.
Good friends understand the importance of each other. To have friends you need to be a good friend.
Friendships don't stay alive or even develop without input from both sides. Sometimes it's easy to take our friends for granted, assuming they will always be there when we need them. A true friend always will be, but take the time to show your appreciation, whether it's a simple phone call at the end of the day to see how they are, or a full-blown dinner party in their honour. They deserve to know just how important they are in your life.

Why don't you spend a while thinking about who your friends are and the influence they have on your life. Are your relationships fairly evenly balanced or do you feel you are doing all the work and putting in all the time. If so, it might be time to back off and cultivate other friendships instead.

Some people are perfectly happy to have a few close and loyal friends, while others thrive best when friends are everywhere and are numerous.

We are all different and we all need different things from friendships. Either way don't ever take them for granted and value the relationship you have with them.

Make The Time For Friends

Always make time for your friends, enjoy their company and make them feel special. You don't need to wait for a special occasion to treat them to lunch or buy a thoughtful small gift. Don't expect anything in return, just treat them well and let them know how much you appreciate them being in your life.

Things To Do With Friends

Time is a precious commodity for most people, so just making 'the time' for your friends is one of the most valuable things you can do.

Go For Lunch

Better still invite them over for lunch. Fresh flowers on the table always look nice, tie a ribbon around the napkin and add a small spray of fresh flowers. Keep the food light, healthy and nutritious. Prepare what you can in advance so you are not busy cooking when you should be chatting. With good friends, good conversation comes easy, but it is always nice to see that an effort has been made for their arrival.

Spa Day

A day at a spa is a nice change from having coffee in the shopping mall, and sometimes you deserve to just treat yourself. It's quite nice to go and just opt for a couple of treatments and spend the rest of the day chatting in your robes in that intoxicating relaxing atmosphere you only get in spas.

Numerologist

If you're into psychics, fortune tellers and the like, why not try a numerologist. Numbers play an important part in your daily lives and certain numbers could be more beneficial to you than others. Invite a few friend's over, have a numerologist come to your home, lay out a few nibbles and drinks and compare numbers!

Join an Evening Class

Learn something new together - it's great for exercising the brain, and is also a good excuse to spend time together, whether it's creative writing, drawing, pottery, pole dancing(who says you're too old!) or wine appreciation. Have a look at what's going on in the area.

Exercise/Gym
Always a good one if you find it hard to motivate yourself to exercise. A bit of moral support will get you going and you will be less likely to quit when the going gets tough.

Call Them
You don't need a reason.

Unexpected Gift
A gift is always nice, especially an unexpected gift. It doesn't have to be expensive, just thoughtful.

Picnic
Always good fun especially if you all have children/grandchildren, and if it rains have it indoors.

Friendship Day - 1st Sunday of August

Happiness

If we could buy it in a bottle, it would be a best seller. We all strive for happiness in our lives, and why wouldn't we? When we are happy we have an inner beauty that shines through and gives us a radiance that no jar of cream ever can, no matter how expensive.

Of course, happiness can mean different things to different people, but one of the main things that distinguishes happy people from unhappy people is their attitude. They have a different way of thinking about things and doing things. They interpret the world in a different way and go about their lives looking at things from a different view point.

What Happiness Isn't
Happiness is not something that comes to you. It is something that you create yourself. Waiting for something to change in order to be happy is like waiting to live your life , and happiness really isn't about having lots of money or being physically attractive or having the latest gadgets. It isn't about acting like a clown, laughing all the while or being at Disneyland having a good time.

So What Is Happiness?
Happiness is a state of mind, well at least 40 percent of it is. Some experts believe that 50 percent of your happiness is genetically determined, so, if your parents are generally happy people chances are you are too. About 10 percent of happiness is dictated by your life circumstances and the remaining 40 percent really is the result of your choices. But don't worry if you didn't do too well in the 'happiness gene pool' because, according to the research, we can still train ourselves to be more content.

It's not what happens to you that counts, it's how you react to what happens to you. When we are presented with problems we need to try and keep things in perspective and remind ourselves of their insignificance in the great scheme of life.

When you have a positive attitude life becomes a rewarding adventure instead of something to get through. The real source of happiness lies within the mind and not in external conditions, and this is something we actually have control over. If something is not right in your life change it, don't spend hours, days, weeks worrying about it all, because nothing will happen until you make that change. Remember you don't find happiness, you make it.

Get a Life: Have an Attitude of Gratitude
Notice the sky full of stars, appreciate the sunny day, enjoy the autumn leaves, pay attention to someone who loves you. Get a life where you are generous, send an e-mail to an old friend, offer a kind gesture to someone, look at the moon in the sky, smell the flowers and appreciate their beauty. Simple pleasures can offer great rewards if you remember to take the time to stop, look and listen.

Benefits Of Laughter
Laughter reduces the level of stress hormones like cortisol and dopamine and increases the level of health enhancing hormones like endorphins and neurotransmitters, which provide an overall sense of well-being.
Laughter provides a physical and emotional release; it strengthens the immune system, reduces stress hormones, boosts energy levels and increases blood flow, which can help protect you against heart attacks and other cardiovascular problems. So for the sake of your health, the next time you find yourself being taken over by what seems to be an awful problem, ask yourself these questions:

Is it really worth getting upset over?
This time next week/month/year will it really matter?
Is it really that important?
Is it really that bad?
Is it really that difficult to fix the problem?
Is it really your problem?

For more inspiration on the art of happiness check out
www.internationalhappinessday.com

Remember that all you experience as a thought is only a thought, and that you are the master of what you think.

Now ask yourself why you would want to live your life always thinking negative thoughts that make you more unhappy?

You are the one who is in control and you are capable of replacing these thoughts with positive, life-loving thoughts, regardless of what you have been through in life.

Final Word

Well, that's it ladies, we have come to the end of our journey but before we say goodbye, just a final few words on HRT…

Humour Replacement Therapy for the Menopause!

Studies carried out on the effects of laughter and the immune system show that laughter lowers blood pressure, reduces stress hormones, increases muscle flexion, and boosts the immune system. That's because laughter triggers the release of endorphins which are the body's natural painkillers.

Humour makes you laugh and laughter makes your body healthier and helps you keep your sanity. If you can see menopause with some humour you'll have a much easier time getting through it.

This form of HRT definitely carries no health warnings with it.

Women's Wisdom

• One of the mysteries of life is that a two pound box of chocolates can make you gain five pounds.
• The reason women over 50 don't have babies is because we would put them down and forget where we put them.
• What happens if you confuse your Valium with your birth control pills?
You have 12 kids, but you don't really care.
• Skinny people annoy me. They say things like, "Sometimes I forget to eat." Now, I've forgotten my keys, my glasses, my pin number and my mother's maiden name. But I have never ever forgotten to eat! You have to be a special kind of stupid to forget to eat!
• My mind doesn't wander, it leaves completely.
• What happens when you leave an outfit hanging in your wardrobe for a while? It shrinks two sizes.
• It's nice to live in a small town, because if you don't know what you are doing, someone else does.

• I read an article which said that the symptoms of stress are impulse buying, eating too much and driving too fast. Are they kidding? That's what I call a perfect day.
• I went to a bookstore and asked the saleswoman, "Where's the self-help section?" She said if she told me, it would defeat the purpose.
• What do you do when you see an endangered animal eating an endangered plant?
• Women are crazy. Men are stupid. The main reason women are crazy is that men are stupid.
• God made man before woman so the man would have time to think of an answer for the woman's first question.

The Real Definition of Words When Used By Women

1. Fine - I am right. This argument is over. You need to shut up.
2. That's okay - One of the most dangerous statements a woman can make to a man. "That's okay" means she wants to think hard and long before deciding when and how you'll pay for your mistake.
3. Nothing - The calm before the storm. This means "something" and you better be on your toes. Note: Arguments that start with "nothing" usually end with "fine" (See #1).
4. Five Minutes - If getting dressed, this means half an hour. (Don't be mad about this. It's the same definition for you when it's your turn to do some chores around the house).
5. Thanks - A woman is thanking you. Do not question this or faint. Just say, "You're welcome," and let it go.
6. Loud Sigh - Not actually a word but rather a non-verbal statement often misunderstood by men. It means she thinks you are an idiot and wonders why she is standing here wasting her time arguing with you about "nothing" (See #3).
7. Go Ahead - This is a dare, not permission. (Don't Do It!).
8. Don't worry about it, I got it - The second most dangerous statement a woman can make. It means that a woman has asked a man several times to do something and is now doing it herself. (This will result in you asking at a later date, "What's wrong?" For the woman's response, see #3).

Differences Between Men and Women

• If Mary, Susan, Claire and Barbara go out for lunch, they will call each other Mary, Susan, Claire and Barbara.
• If John, Mark, Tony and Daniel go out, they will affectionately refer to each other as Bruno, Scrappy, Peanut-Head and Godzilla.
• A man has five items in his bathroom: a toothbrush, razor, shaving cream, a bar of soap, and a towel.
• The average number of items in a woman's bathroom is 328. The average man would not be able to identify most of them.
• Women always have the last word in an argument. Anything a man adds after that is the beginning of a new argument.
• A woman worries about the future -- until she gets a husband.
• A successful man is one who makes more money than can be spent by his wife.
A successful woman is one who can find that man.
• A woman marries a man expecting he will change, but he doesn't. A man marries a woman expecting that she won't change, and she does.
• Men wake up looking as good as when they went to bed. Women somehow deteriorate during the night.
• A woman knows all about her children. She knows about their best friends, romances, secret hopes and dreams, favourite foods, fears and dental appointments.
A man is vaguely aware of some short people living in the house.
• Married men should forget their mistakes. There is no need for two people to remember the same thing.

Why Men Are Happier

• Men can play with toys all their life.
• Men can wear shorts no matter what their legs look like.
• Men have one wallet and one pair of shoes which are good for every season.
• Men can choose whether or not to grow a moustache.
• Men can "do" their fingernails with a pocket knife.
• Men's bellies usually hide their large hips.
• Chocolate is just another snack.
• The whole garage belongs to them.

- Everything on a man's face stays its original colour.
- Men only have to shave their faces and necks.
- Men can keep the same hairstyle for years, even decades.
- Men can do their Christmas shopping for 25 relatives on Christmas Eve in 25 minutes.
- For men, wrinkles add character.
- Men can go on a week's vacation and pack only one suitcase.
- Men's new shoes don't cause blisters, or cut or mangle their feet.
- Men don't have to stop and think which way to turn a screw.
- Men have one mood all the time.
- Men can open all their own jars.

The Last laugh

After being married 25 years, a man looked at his wife one day and said, "You know, 25 years ago we lived in a cheap apartment, drove a cheap car, had only a sofa bed and watched a 14" black and white television. BUT, every night I got to sleep with a hot 25 year old blonde."
Now,"he continued", we have a nice house, a new car, a big flat-screen TV, but I have to sleep with a 50 year old woman. It doesn't seem fair."
His wife was a reasonable woman. She replied, "Well, why don't you go out and get yourself a hot 25 year old blonde? Then I'll make sure you will once again live in a cheap apartment, drive a cheap car, have only a sofa bed and watch a 14" black and white television."

The man rethought his priorities.

• (not) The End
Your New Beginning xx

Index

A

B

C

D

E

F

Folic acid, 42
Follicile stimulating hormone, 29
Foods groups, 119
Foot
    spa ritual, 197
Free radicals
    skin changes, 47
Fruits, 13

G

Ginkgo biloba, 35
Ginseng, 39, 74
Glucose
    and insulin resistance, 110
Gomasio, 154, 155
Good fats
    and bad fats, 133
Gotu Kola, 40, 75

H

Hair
    and testosterone, 28
    and top 10 foods, 184
    facial, 185
    pubic, 51
Hand
    massage, 201
Hands
    care ritual, 200
Happiness, 247
Headache
    & Migrains, 42
Heart
    diseases, 63
Heart disease, 72, 84, 100, 112, 129, 131, 133, 134, 139, 141, 144, 145, 149, 161
Heart rate, 83
Herbal remedies, 225
Herbs
    bath bags, 189
Hirsutism, 47
Homeopathy, 76
Hormone
    and levels, 11
    and tests, 10
    estrogen, 17
    imbalance, 14

I

J

Milk Baths, 190
Minerals
 - for the skin, 174
Mitochondria, 13
Monounsaturated Fats, 132
Mood Swings, 33
Muscle
 - face exercise, 101
 - fast twitch and slow twitch, 86
 - Major Groups, 87
 and BMI, 117
 and calcium, 150
 and magnesium, 150
 -benefits of exercise, 81
 exercise, 85
 -tension, 45

N

Nails, 137, 149, 198
Night Sweats, 31

O

Oestrogen
 and anxiety, 41
 and bone health, 55
 and cancer, 20
 and creams, 171
 and depression, 34
 and HRT, 60
 and joint pain, 44
 and loss of libido, 51
 and memory loss, 38
 and mood swings, 33
 and phytomone spa therapy, 35
 and skin changes, 46
 and sleep problems, 36
 and tender breasts, 48
 and urinary tract problems, 49
 and weight gain, 32
 Female Sex hormones, 13
 Hormone tests, 10
 hot flushes, 29
 Menopause, 11
 Post menopause, 12
 why we gain weight, 108
Omega, 39, 44, 47, 48, 73, 130, 131, 132, 144, 184

Osteoporosis, 12, 55, 56, 61, 72, 75, 77, 84, 87, 159
Ovaries
   - unresponsive, 10
   and FSH, 15
   and hormones, 12
Ovulation, 10, 24, 25, 51
Oxalic acid, 57

P

Pain
   - joint, 20
   -breasts, 26
   -in chest, 42
   -in joints, 43
Pelvic Floor Exercises, 93
Pelvic floor muscles, 93
Perfect Pampering, 186
Peri-menopause, 10, 12, 14, 17, 28, 32, 42, 44, 66, 69, 70, 74
Physiological Benefits
   -meditation, 210
Phyto-oestrogens, 7, 24, 50, 51, 138, 142, 144
Pilates, 55, 87, 88, 89
Polycystic ovaries, 19
Polyunsaturated fats, 130
Post Menopause, 12
pregnancy, 24, 25, 75
Pregnancy, 15, 17
Progesterone
   and HRT, 60
   and levels, 24
   -bio identical, 25
   -cream, 31
   -Deficiency, 27
   -Dominance, 27
   -natural, 25
   -progestins, 26
   -progestogens, 26
Protein
   -choosing the right soy, 138
   -good for and bad for, 138
   -good sources, 137
   -requirements, 137
Psychological
   -benifits meditation, 210

R

Recipe
   -Body scrub, 195
   -Gomasio, 154
   -Hand massage oil, 201
Red Clover, 75
Reflexology, 76
Relaxation, 191, 201, 210, 211, 215
Restless legs, 35, 39
Rheumatoid Arthritis, 72
Running, 89

S

Sage, 74
Salt
   -healthy substitute, 153
   -leaching of calcium, 58
   requirements, 152
   -scrubs, 194
Seaweed, 40
   and kelp, 144
Senses
   -sensuous living, 231
Sensuality
   in the bedroom, 232
Sex
   and ginseng, 74
   -feeling sexy again, 52
   -loss of libido, 51
   sexiest essential oils, 236
   Tantric sex, 233
Skeleton, 54
Skin
   -Ageing, 168
   -anti-ageing creams, 170
   -bathing, 188
   body moisturizers, 196
   -botox, 177
   -care, 166
   care regime, 169
   -changes in menopause, 46
   -dry body brushing, 192
   -estrogen cream, 171
   Hand care, 199
   Happy feet, 196
   -home facial, 175

X

Y

Z

We hope you enjoyed "The Menopause Secret"
Are you ready to make the change for "The Change"?
Then invest in -
"The Menopause 30 Day Concierge Programme"
ISBN:978-1477534991

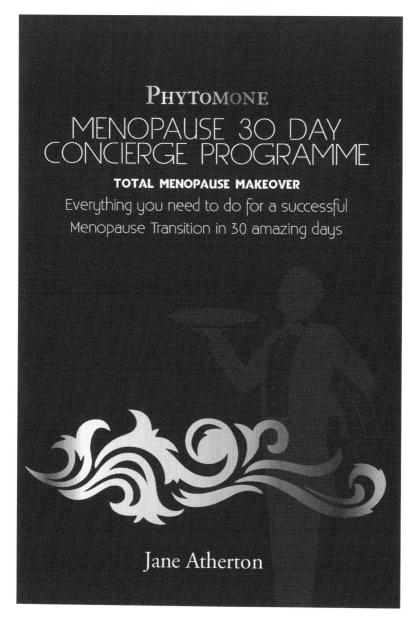

Made in the USA
Charleston, SC
13 November 2013